To Gail

THE FOOTPRINTS OF FUNNY FEET

Always keep the remotes handy.

THE FOOTPRINTS OF FUNNY FEET

Anthony Sicilia

Copyright © 2022 by Anthony Sicilia

All rights reserved

No part of this book may be reproduced, stored in a retrieval system, or transmitted by any means, electronic, mechanical, photocopying, recording, or otherwise, without written permission from the author or publisher. There is one exception. Brief passages may be quoted in articles or reviews.

Library and Archives Canada Cataloguing in Publication

CIP data on file with the National Library and Archives

ISBN 978-1-55483-502-7

To my nieces Angelina, Nora and Sianna
(I love you)

To my beloved nieces Angelina, Nora and Sianna. This book is dedicated to you three when Daddy becomes too old to read you a bedtime story. These pages must be read to the girls to understand how to react to a person with special needs. Whenever they see someone different from them, I would ask that the girls judge a person's character. Even if that person has a bad character, continue to show love, empathy, and kindness even if the same is not returned to you. Love always conquers... Remember that...

Table of Contents

	Prologue for Pundits	9
1.	The Blue Faced Baby	11
2.	The Origins of Funny Feet	15
3.	Mom & Dad deal with my funny feet in two very different ways	17
4.	The Fears of My Peers a Foreword by Nathan Innes	21
5.	Unable to WRITE Makes Me a perfect candidate to TYPE	26
6.	The Good and Bad Guys of Television	28
7.	View From Outside the Pine Box	32
8.	A Very Special Olympic History	36
9.	Bed Pans and Bad Food	38
10.	A Protein Shake and A Weight Room	40
11.	The Pen is Mightier than the sword — The Journalism Years	43
12.	Climbing Mount Olympus Without Leaving My Backyard	45
13.	Caught Between the Ropes Chasing A Lion's Tale, The Ray Barone Life	48
14.	There is ACTION in Akron	51
15.	Going to Bible College on a Greyhound	54
16.	Help, A Hard Thing For a Man to Ask	59
17.	Ulcers and Ambulance Rides	63
18.	Happy Days with Hiatal Hernia	66
19.	Parkwood Prison	72
20.	A New Hip at 36	77
21.	Doctors of Doubt Disabling Your Rights	80
22.	Tenacity in Toronto	86
23.	These Bones Can Live!	88
24.	Clark Kent's Swan Song	90
	Acknowledgments	94

Prologue For Pundits

I am going to keep this entry chapter real short and sweet. Down through the years, there have been a variety of books, movies and television series about the disability of Cerebral Palsy. However, the one thing many people fail to realize is that there are various types of CP. Along with there being different types of the same disability, there are different categories, but many people fail to acknowledge that. Due to their failure to acknowledge specialized and specific treatments, all people with the condition known as Cerebral Palsy get lumped under one stigma. We're all either crippled or (handicapped). Let me be honest, so my readers understand that we **hate** being called **crippled.** Calling someone with our deformity crippled is like calling Marty McFly a chicken or yellow belly. It's just a bad choice of words unless you are looking for a fight. My advice for a generation of normal feet is to be more compassionate to someone struggling but not be overbearing or think that people with physical disabilities are entirely useless...

CHAPTER 1
The Blue Faced Baby

The day of my birth will not be written in the scientific Journal, Time magazine, National Geographic or the New York times, even though I think it should be because the circumstances behind how I came to earth was anything but normal. I was born the second child of four, but even more impressive is that I didn't come alone; I have a twin brother. My siblings are as follows in chronological order (Michael was born in April 1981, my twin brother Angelo was born in May 1985,

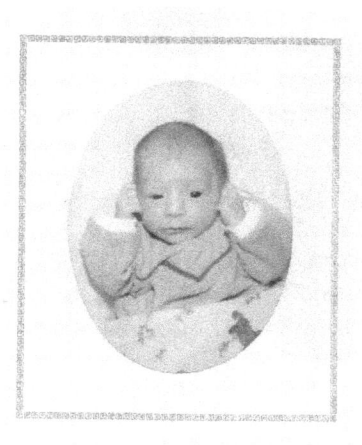

(Little Anthony) 8 months old

and my younger sibling Sara was born in April 1988. Here's a little bit of truth. Aside from my twin brother Angelo, I have no idea how I and the other siblings are related as we have absolutely nothing in common and don't even speak. My older brother Michael and my younger sister Sara might as well be Aliens in our family. However, they both have one thing about them that I completely detest. Michael and Sara both have an arrogant sense of entitlement to their attitude.

Perhaps that is the answer to the $250,000 question about why we seem so distant from one another. Angelo was the closest person to me because he arrived on the scene born just

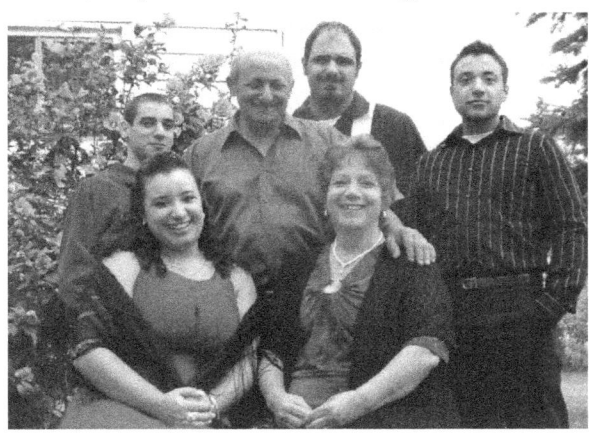

Family photo outside our St. Marys Farm House. August 2012

— 11 —

3 ½ minutes after I was. I poke fun at the time difference and being older, but it doesn't seem to bother him because he's taller. The date was May 26, 1985. It seems so long ago now that it almost feels like ancient history. Although I declared my birth was nothing special, the hospital realized that I did require immediate medical attention after a health scare.

I required a defibrillator to stay alive. That's right, the first moments of my birth were breathtaking because it took my breath away, and that's a fact. The reasons behind losing oxygen while placed in an incubator are still bewilderment or strange incident to medical experts studying the condition of cerebral palsy. After discovering that I had the condition now known as CP, my parents were in shock.

I'm sure they wanted to express a different emotion other than anger. They should have been happy, after all, they gave birth to twins. Although contrary to popular belief, I started as a normal baby, born seven weeks premature on May 26, 1985, at 3 pounds and 13 ounces. My twin brother Angelo was born 3 minutes after I was; he was 3 pounds at birth. I still bother my brother about being older than him, but he is taller and has more hair. However, I'm the more robust type. I'm convinced my brother and I fought in the womb-like Jacob and Esau.

I say I was born normal, and that is entirely true. The circumstances of how I developed cerebral palsy occurred after my birth when I was placed in an incubator without an oxygen tank. Now I'm no medical doctor or anything, but I think if you place a baby who is prematurely born in an incubator without any oxygen, that isn't good. Even though I developed CP moments after my birth, ordinary things weren't meant to happen on that day. My twin brother Angelo happened to develop asthma, and as a result, he had breathing problems.

On the same day of giving birth to my brother and me, my mother discovered she was born with one kidney. Boy, when they say bad things happen in threes, it sometimes does, and that's only the surface. It would take some time for doctors to determine that I had cerebral palsy because for me to get diagnosed, I needed to walk, and I wasn't walking until I was eleven months.

When my father walked into the room where I was lying and

saw that my face turned blue, he wanted to grab every nurse in the place and smash their head against a wall. After being told by the doctor that I would have Cerebral Palsy, my parents wanted to sue St. Joseph's Hospital for malpractice, but after talking to a few doctors in the family overseas in Italy, they convinced my mother and father not to sue the hospital because of the time and stress that would be involved in the task.

My cousin convinced my father to focus specifically on my physical needs like specialized therapy to quell my father's outrage. There was only one problem: I lived in Canada, even though health care is "free" after paying your taxes.

Physical therapy for a small child who just wants to be like every other boy can be challenging. If I was being completely honest when it came to therapy, I hated it, because it took me away from what I thought were more important things in life at the time like playing Super Mario Bros on the Nintendo. Because of that, my father and mother would face a vast array of challenges in seeking out specialists, physical therapists and nutrition experts.

According to medical experts, my parents did the best they could with what they had to work with, which wasn't much. I was very blessed in one aspect of my physical condition because it could have been worse. I could have been required to be in a wheelchair or bedridden for the remainder of my natural life. However, circumstances beyond my control ensured that I wouldn't have a difficult life like those described in books and movies...

The dedication that my parents showed to my illness would mark them commendable. As much as I had to battle with doing things a bit differently physically, they had to fight with the mental aspect of getting me well enough to lead a normal life.

> "Therefore, I take pleasure in infirmities, in reproaches, in necessities, in persecutions, in distresses for Christ's sake: for when I am weak, then am I strong," 2 Corinthians 12:10.

I believe that is why they strived so hard because they wanted to spare me getting teased. The courage and strength showcased by my parents during my early years would give me the initiative and drive to keep going. Learning how to do things differently from other kids didn't always come easy to me, and I was always looked at as being a bit weird for going against the norm.

Some of you might think that just because I had a physical disability, everyone and everything was made a bit easier for me; not so, at that time, I was the only one who had a disability. Nothing and no one made things easier for me; you may ask yourselves the question why, and I have the perfect answer for that. Nothing in life was made easier for me because people who had issues with their mental capacity and physical dilemmas at the time were few and far between. They were not as noticeable. Instead of having the school conform to my needs, I had to conform to the school. I believe this is why I have the drive and determination I do because I had to deal with many barriers and obstacles.

Doctors can have 30 different medical diplomas, but they will not begin to understand what it is like for parents to hear devastating news about their child's health. At the time of the announcement of my health issues, my parents were experiencing bouts of frustration, anger and overall wonder about whether or not they had the strength to raise a child with his physical condition that requires so much attention. I spent the majority of my early years outside of school.

How I passed elementary school, considering the number of days I missed, is beyond my comprehension. Many people would consider my road trips to hospitals fun because they got me out of school; let me ask my readers: What makes travelling to the hospital to see doctors and nurses fun?

Waiting on a doctor is a lot like waiting on dial-up internet.

You're always waiting for someone, and while you're sitting in the waiting room, you, the patient, are trying to keep yourself entertained before the expert or surgeon walks through the door.

Most of the time, these doctors examined my motion; the doctors would often have me X-rayed and ask me many questions to which I knew no answer.

That being said, I did enjoy eating a pizza while on the road, when this kind of thing happened to me, I felt spoiled. "Oh, what a simple life I led as a small child that eating a pizza while taking a day off school mattered so much to me then."

CHAPTER 2
The Origins of My Funny Feet

This chapter gives the readers insight into why I thought writing this book became an essential part of telling my story. So that everyone understands that this chapter is based on various experiences, and it includes being inspired by a multitude of people. In other words, aside from talking about how I began to name this book, there are several people that I have met or have been inspired by that formulated the book you are currently reading.

If I am frank with you, a book like this wouldn't even be possible without technology because the deformity has made my printing and penmanship comparable to the chicken scratch of a doctor's note. As a child, my printing was so terrible that my primary school French teacher thought I had dyslexia. There are a group of teachers in my college years to that I owe a debt of gratitude. Writing a book like this would not have even come close to just being a pipe dream without their guidance. Without their understanding and endless patience with me and my literacy shortcomings, they as a collective team are the real reason why I am even remotely able to string a single paragraph together and make sense of it all...

This book is possible because of Norman Pearson's 1989 film My Left Foot, starring Daniel Day-Lewis, Hugh O'Conor and Brenda Fricker. Growing up, my parents made me watch the movie every year as a small child, and after watching the film, they left me with a resounding message. "Anthony, why can't you be like Christy Brown? He used one foot and look at the success he became."After years of thinking about it, my rebuttal is, Mom and Dad: There are different types of cerebral palsy, and we, as people who are disabled, shouldn't be lumped in with the lot. If my parents believe that the movie of My Left Foot inspires their lives, that's great, but to say that Christy Brown, the painter, the author, never experienced struggle is far beyond a misunderstanding. One of the significant reasons I wanted to write a book like this is to show the audience of my readers that I don't want to live by the stigmas of being labelled as a useless crippled; I want to break down barriers. The beginning steps in doing that happen by writing this book.

CHAPTER 3

My Mother and Father deal with my Funny Feet in two very different ways

Growing up, I was given two types of parental teams: a no-nonsense father and a complex compassionate mother. I compare my father's outlook on life as the former **Roman Emperor Nero and Italian dictator Mussolini** rolled into one. These days if interviewed, I am sure Mom and Dad would agree that they showed me love. They will openly talk about how they made sacrifices because I was the centre of their love, and they will openly admit that I was deeply loved, well above my other three siblings. If anyone has met them and believes their perspective, then I hate to be the one to burst your bubble of being gullible.

I spent the early years of my childhood afraid to go to sleep. As a youngster, I battled insomnia from ages nine to 22. The reason is that I didn't know what type of father I would get from day to day. I often believed that my father had two personalities, and the most common two personalities I can think of is the Dr. Jekyll and Mr. Hyde.

Make no mistake about it; I love my family for what they have done for me. My mother is a lady that cooked so much food that it became her way of showing a sense of appreciation to people. On the other hand, my father was rigorous. He was the disciplinarian in the family.

Often my parents and I were going here, there, and everywhere to find solutions to what some would consider complex medical conditions. I am fairly sure that sometimes if my father would STOP and turn his attention to God for answers regarding how best to handle situations, he would have been able to use more wisdom beyond human comprehension. By doing that, he could have more confidence in what he was doing, and I know for sure that if my parents clutched the Bible to their chest and read it as most should, I'm under the assumption that they could have saved themselves a lot of heartaches, headaches, and heart attacks. Sometimes, as human beings rely on what our eyes see as simple truth. However, I know from experience that you should never look at a glass being half empty. In our human experiences as people, we can sometimes fail to see that God is in control.

I do not doubt that as parents, some of the decisions they had to make were tough, but if they wanted peace, comfort, love and understanding, they could have found that solace in the scriptures.

The kindest thing I can say about my childhood is that I survived it. When I say that my mother and emperor Nero dealt with me having CP in two very different ways, that's exactly what I mean, and I'm not sugar coding anything. My mother spent most of her life walking around how she could be home for me when I came home from school—making my lunches. Helping me study and even doing physical exercises and games with me, I would be interested in maintaining some sort of normal walking gait. However, emperor Nero chose to deal with my cerebral palsy in a way that made him drink continuously, starting in the early morning with shots of brandy before going to work as a mason—then coming home for lunch, finishing off a bottle of wine and then going back to work. He would start a bottle of wine at supper and finish it in one sitting. He was and will always be a drunk, and that isn't a real good father. That's a man who's lost his way along with various brain cells because it is excessive drinking.

Emperor Nero couldn't handle having a son with CP so much whenever I couldn't do anything physically because of my disability. I was whipped and beaten profusely until my father was satisfied after seeing the sight of blood from my eyes or nose.

My mother spent her precious time trying to give me a life that wouldn't seem unorthodox my father was never satisfied with my physical condition and became very angry because of that. I was counted as worthless and useless because I could not be a stonemason like my father or brothers. My father's temperament came into play; I was the source of all his rage because of a disability. I spent most of my early childhood years going to appointment after an appointment four days a week at Thames Valley Children

Centre. I always loved going to appointments with my mother but hated going with my father, or emperor Nero, as I call him. Whenever I went to doctors' appointments with emperor Nero in the driver's seat, he would constantly belittle me about how I should be better physically, and I had a genuine attitude problem because I wasn't listening to him and his divine instruction referred to it as.

My mother dealt with me very tenderly, she knew I didn't want to be at these various doctor's appointments. She knew deep down all I wanted to do was be like everyone other kid who gets to play with his friends and from time to time perhaps if I was fortunate enough, I could maybe have an opportunity to drink chocolate milk. My parents received a small inheritance from the government because they had a child with cerebral palsy. When my mother got ahold of this money, she used it for good purposes like buying groceries or spending money on clothes and shoes for school. When my father got access to this money, he built a hot tub—an extra bathroom in a huge bedroom. I don't see how having an additional big bedroom benefits me at all. My parent's inheritance given to them by the government also allowed them to use some of the money for my doctor's appointments when paying for gas. I always hated going to doctors' appointments with my father because Nero always stated that I took food off his table with every doctor's appointment that I went to.

The relationship I had with Emperor Nero deteriorated from day one. He didn't like to have a son with a disability because it made him look weak, and in the public eye, because he was a well-known Mason, he didn't want to look weak. My mother had her moments, but at the end of the day, my mother was a SAINT for the sacrifices she had to endure being married to Emperor Nero. I'm sure it was no easy task. My mom sacrificed so much, but even before I shared my educational tour, she wanted to make sure I had every advantage, so she made sure that she left no stone unturned. She would make sure I would go to speech therapy. She would make sure that I had an excellent printing ability, but I had an excellent medical set team around me that included a physical therapist who would come into the schools.

She ensured that I would have a good occupational therapist who would work with me on my speech and printing ability, which would pay dividends because I would become a journalist as a major in college. My mother is, was, and will always be a SAINT.

CHAPTER 4
The Fears of my Peers
A FOREWORD BY NATHAN INNES

I'd love to take this time to tell you all about my good friend Anthony, but after reading his life story, I feel he doesn't leave much to say. I think I can give some perspective and some validation to this inspiring tale. The best example is to take you back to the first day I met Anthony over two decades ago.

I attended a small rural public school. Quaint and not accustomed to out-of-the-ordinary happenings. It was grade two near the beginning of the year. Alliances and friends began to emerge, and our multiplication tables were practiced daily.

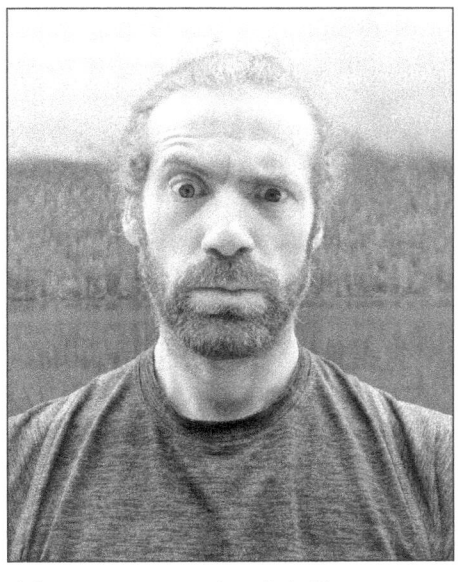

The day Anthony and his brother Angelo arrived was one I can still see vividly in my mind. I came to school as usual and began speaking to my best friend, Ryan.

Suddenly, a grey platform was ushered in through the door, followed by someone carrying a padded wooden chair. They set it at the front of the class, right next to the blackboard. First, they placed the grey platform down. It had holes in it where they secured the legs of the chair into. The chair even had Velcro straps on it for support of some kind.

However, as a child, it looked like some kind of chair used for punishment. Then moments later, Anthony walked in. I had never seen anyone with a physical disability before, and I can say, in combination with the punishment chair, I thought Anthony must be uncontrollable! An animal! (I found this out to be accurate but in a much different context, dealing with his perseverance and courage)

However, like most children, my preconceptions didn't invoke fear. It invoked curiosity, and I will forever be grateful for that because it not only set a precedent for how I would grow up and view those who are different, but it gave me the rich opportunity to make a great friend.

Since then, we spent hours at his computer co-writing story after story in our younger years. Even when our proximity wasn't close enough to be at the same computer, we have spent many years in dialogue about the more significant questions in life and have kept in touch to this day.

I have witnessed Anthony go for what he believes in and never let his physical limitations hold him back throughout the years. He is a born storyteller, and I am positive you will enjoy hearing about his journey.

—**Nathan Alexander Innes.**

Now that you know a bit of the background behind my birth, it's about time that I tell you a short story about how my classmates received me in school. I lived in an age in the early '90s where words would become weapons. Both for good purposes and bad. "Sticks and stones will break your bones, but names will never hurt you." That was the motto with which I went to elementary school. I came as a foreigner into this new public school system.

Before entering the public school system for the first time, I was educated in the Christian School System. There I would dress nice, polish my shoes and use way too much gel in my combed hair just to try and look like a 'saint' to my teachers. I spent two years in the Christian school system, only to be removed simply because no physical activities were required for me to move about. Because I would need much physical activity beyond running and playing outside for recess, I was transferred to elementary school in a country where physical education was a class unto itself.

I had never witnessed gym class before. I didn't know what to think. I was just happy I didn't get smashed in the face with a baseball or dodge ball. When I entered elementary school for the first time within the public school system, I was an alien to most students. Nine out of 10 peers inside my classroom were convinced I had a form of leprosy. Because of this, they kept their distance.

I didn't know how much I would stand out until a small child not too much younger than I was at the time would ask me now the infamous question that would transform my life in many different ways. I was age 7 when I entered elementary school, and being on the playground was strange to me, but even more bizarre were the gawking eyes that were led in my direction. I was a very quiet child in school. I kept not causing too much trouble unless trouble came looking for me. The moment I first realized I would stand out from the crowd as easily as a clown on wall street was the moment when a girl named Nancy once asked me a question as I was outside during recess.

She came up to me, and with a weird glare in her eyes and stunning curiosity, she asked me, "Why do you walk so funny?"

The elementary school I attended had never witnessed a person having a physical disability.

Oh, to be the first one wasn't as joyful as one may expect. As the school day ended, the question regarding my physical disability rattled in my brain like an atomic bomb. All I thought why was I so different from the others? What is wrong with me? When I got home, I was determined to investigate and get to the bottom of the whole situation.

I came in the door fuming like a volcano waiting to erupt. I called for my mother. "Mom," I said, "why do I walk so differently from the other kids." As soon as I asked her that question, I could almost read the expression on her face. She said, "I wish I didn't have to tell you this so early on in life; you will not understand yet." She kindly replied, "Go ask your Dad."

Later that night, my dad would turn down the volume on the television to reveal to me that I had a physical disability because of an accident that happened at birth. He said, "I saw your face go blue, and it haunts me to this day." I explained why I had wondered why I walked so funny; he said, kids will pick on you because you are different from them. A few weeks later, my father would begin to teach me about boxing. I was never allowed to use it against anyone unless they caused harm to me first. It was to be used strictly as a form of self-defense. At age nine, I had lightning hand speed. I would practice boxing twice a week and do my physical therapy three times a week.

The nineties ushered in the era of sports and musicals. Guess which ones I took part in; one guess says it wasn't football.... I often tried my best to play with the other kids, but I was that one kid that was picked last for everything and I did everything....

I think this type of favouritism occurs because people sometimes fear what they don't understand. Academically the only challenge I faced in the classroom was the poor penmanship I had; however, technology helped that learning curve. The school I attended pulled their resources together and purchased a computer for me for in-class assignments. When the school bought a laptop for me, I took to that piece of technology like a fish swimming in the water. Also, I took up writing and reading more often. I always enjoyed reading and writing; I used to write many a story, and I used it as a way for me to escape my everyday life.

As I began to read and write, I started to understand words. Because I had developed a more profound understanding of words, my imagination was used to transport me inside the pages of any book I was reading. Two of my favourite authors were Robert Munsch and Roald Dahl as a child. When I first read the book Charlie and The Chocolate Factory, I fell in love with chocolate and still, after all these years, I still love chocolate; it all began with a simple children's book. Unlike my dislike for pancakes, and yes, if we have time, I will explain to my readers why I dislike pancakes a little later in the book.

I first began writing stories when I was just nine years old, and it's fascinating that 21 years later, I am still writing; the only thing that has changed is the things I read. As I said earlier, I am quite interested in history, and I believe that is why these days, I could spend many days in God's Word studying it and constantly learning. Here's an important fact to remember, whether you have a high school, college or even university diploma, it's essential always to maintain a love for knowledge. I do that by spending hours speaking the scriptures written in my textbooks, and it's truly a beautiful thing. I will say that even though my peers who look only with their physical eyes see my disability as a stumbling block to them, I beg to differ.

I was only crippled and disabled when I didn't serve God with my whole being, mind, body and soul.... I still have a passion for writing, but it should be understood that even though I had a passion for writing, I didn't always have the precision with punction that I do today.

I have a good understanding of writing now because I had a wonderful college professor, and I'm sure I taught him the value of long-suffering. I say this because my writing style was awful; I never went by the book. I always created my own path, and if it weren't for my college professors believing in my creative passion, I wouldn't be half the writer I am today. I will tell you the truth, being unable to write legibly made me the perfect candidate to type, and I have just never really stopped. I had a passion for writing but early on in my writing days I didn't always have the precision with punctuation that I do today. I just needed help to mold me into a writer that people could understand. As a child, I could take stories that I read and transform them into my vision, whether it was changing the beginning, middle or end. Writing stories was exciting, but like all good aspiring writers, I needed help. So, I put together a team of friends that kept me on track and in line to create the perfect formula for a good story.

CHAPTER 5
Unable to WRITE makes me a perfect candidate to TYPE

Initially, this chapter was a write-off, but later in the writing process, I realized how essential a chapter like this would be to the book's existence. The reason I felt a chapter like this would be necessary for the overall finished product of the book is that having cerebral palsy and dealing with surgeries and more surgeries is one thing, but when I got Cerebral Palsy, most people, if they are not paying attention only see the diagnosis of CP as simply a physical limitation and barrier only for the legs. However, there is more to the disability than just that. Cerebral Palsy also affects the hands and arms in some instances. Most of the time, it just means the limbs won't be able to stretch out without medical assistance. That's why certain professions exist, like occupational therapy and physical therapy. The use of physical therapy allows limbs to be stretched and strengthened. Whereas occupational therapy allows a person to be well acquainted with needs in the home or school.

An example of this is perhaps they need a unique chair to assist with the straightening of the spine; maybe they need to work on their printing and writing ability. Perhaps they need specific computer programs to be well versed for their years in school to have the same educational advantages as everyone else. When we discovered I had CP, I originally didn't want anything to change because I didn't want to be labelled or typecast from a group of classmates in a certain way. After a while, the more I grew up, the more I realized that I had a problem writing.

When some of my teachers ripped up my reports for being illegible, even though it wasn't my fault. Some of my early teachers thought I was writing to garner sympathy for grades. For most of my early years in school, the teachers always thought one-dimensional. They knew that Cerebral Palsy affected the limbs, but in no way did they think that there would also be a limitation or barrier in my arms, which would make writing and printing for me very difficult. It wasn't until I entered fourth grade that my teachers had a very private meeting about effectively getting me to communicate legibly. In fourth grade, I would utilize the assistance of an IBM computer to get my school and classroom assignments done.

Meanwhile, if I had to take home my schoolwork, I also had a Commodore 64. Yes, I realize that I'm dating myself, but I'm telling the truth. The real question that everyone wants to know is, with all the technology at home: Did you get straight A's now that everyone could read my writing? The short answer is: No, I didn't. I was far too busy at nine years old playing duck hunt and high noon to ever care about anything to do with school. I used to procrastinate a lot as a kid. In the early years of using a computer, my parents considered the technology a complete waste of time. I have a small message for my mom and Dad; with how technology has advanced in recent years and given your disposition toward new forms of technology, why are you both on Facebook? I guess I won the debate on how useful computers can become if used correctly. There are instances where society has to go with the times.

CHAPTER 6
The Good and Bad Guys of Television

There he was; he was larger-than-life. He was a mega-muscled superhero, and his name was Hulk Hogan. This is the story of how professional wrestling influenced me as a youngster, as a teenager and well into my adult years.

When I first witnessed Hulk Hogan on the television screen, I was seven years old. I'd never seen wrestling before. The first time I saw a wrestling match taking place, I was visiting my grandparents one Saturday afternoon. While my grandfather was in the kitchen preparing his usual meal of spaghetti and meatballs, I was left to channel surf alone. I first watched the red and yellow-wearing wrestler on *Saturday Night's Main Event* on television.

When my grandfather came into the room to tell me, "Anthony, It's time for lunch." He witnessed me watching wrestling. He shook his head he walked over to turn off the TV. Before, we would have an opportunity to say to me to eat lunch. "Nono," as I affectionately called him, proceeded to tell me a story about him from his youth. He told me that he was once a fan of professional wrestling in a time when it had more professionalism rather than it being a three-act play. As my grandfather grew up, he became a super fan.

He even had a favourite wrestler—fellow Italian native Bruno Sammartino. I didn't know what to think because I had no idea who Sammartino was at that time. Nono would tell me how Bruno was the best in his day; he was even a world champion for seven years. A record that still holds up today in wrestling history. My grandfather would tell me that when he became a father, one of his favourite past times as a father would be to take his children to local wrestling matches. One night my grandfather witnessed, to his shock and disappointment, a "pulled punch." Which refers to giving more of a reaction to a punch than actually expressing a sense of real pain. He said that he would never again watch or respect the wrestling business after that. I put my grandfather in a challenging position because when he saw my eyes glowing with excitement after viewing wrestling, he chose to watch wrestling with me on Saturdays rather than disappoint his grandson. What a lovely grandpa he was.

One of the other reasons I also went over there is that going to church was just part of the Italian way. So, our weekends were planned out; Saturdays were reserved for watching wrestling and eating spaghetti, while Sunday was God's time. I can remember stepping inside the Roman Catholic Church and kneeling at the door; I also had to dip my finger in holy water and put a cross on my forehead using the water that I had just dropped my fingers into. I felt strange, and the service didn't even start yet.... I went through this routine for many years, but I wasn't ready to hear the gospel as a young boy. Another reason my grandparents loved having me over at their house was because I paid so much attention to them. I called twice a day up until the day they both died. When I returned home from school, I would turn on the TV to watch the sports highlights, but there were no highlights on, but to my surprise and joy, wrestling was. I was thrilled.

I was excited and couldn't wait to see what would unfold. I did have my favourites, and I even had the wrestlers that would scare me half to death. My favourite wrestlers were the clear fan favourites, but on the other end of the spectrum, characters like Paul Bearer and The Ultimate Warrior would scare me so much that they would take years off my life... Aside from being scared by a few things in wrestling that went bump in the night, I was thrilled to watch such a program. I was blessed the first time I watched wrestling at home because my father wasn't home at that time. My mother caught me watching wrestling, and after she asked how I started watching that. She then called her father, my grandfather, to ask him what he had done to me? My mother knew that her grandfather was a former fan. However, my mother despised pro wrestling. Even more than that, my father was once a famous boxer well known throughout Europe as a boxer. He had a deep passion for the sweet science, and he said no to wrestling.

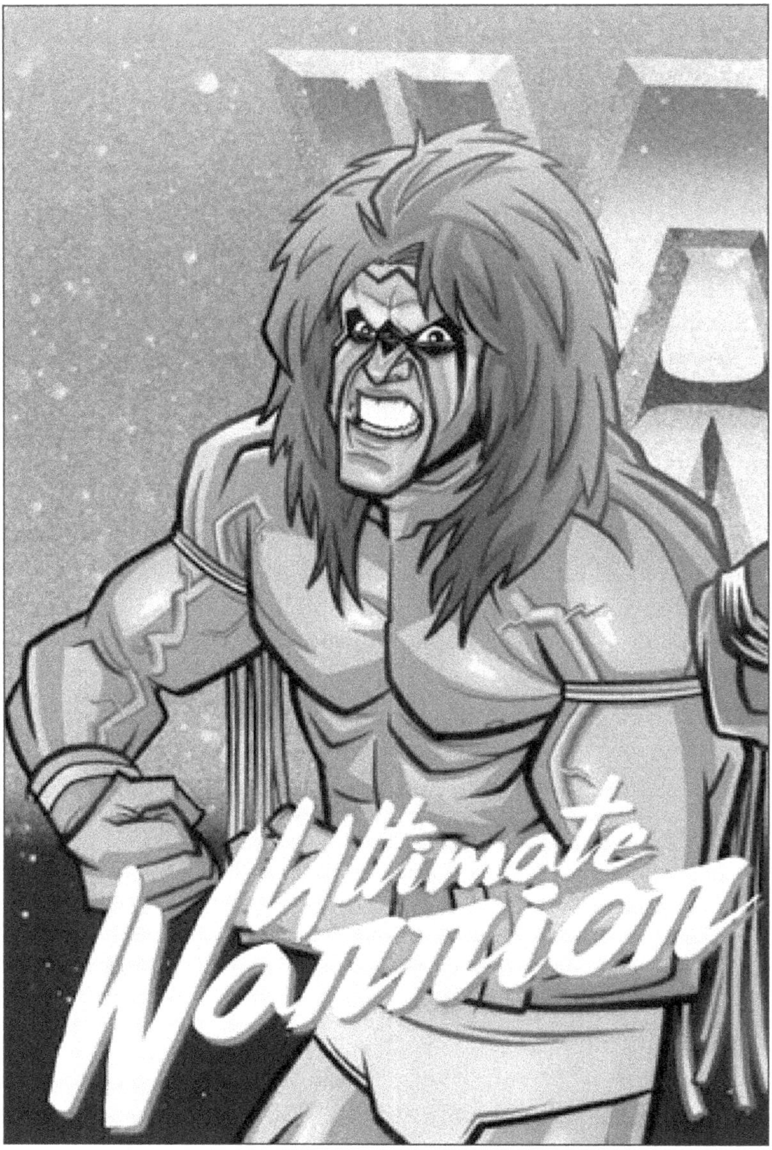
Ultimate
Warrior

My father believed that wrestling was dumb; he also thought the sport of professional wrestling made a mockery of physically fit athletes. This was worse when it was later discovered that many wrestlers looked the way they did through performance enhancers. At the time, I didn't care. I loved the action, drama even the comedy. I was hooked. I was a wrestling fan, and it would be a tough habit to break.

Who were the Good Guys of Television, and what did they do for me? The good guys of TV were men of God. I started tuning into TV ministers because my parents had a spat in a service with one of the members, which discouraged them from attending church regularly, even if it was just two hours away from Detroit. I had to watch good Godly programs in secret because my family thought they didn't need to hear God's word. Their reason behind this way of thinking was that we had a Bible in our home and although we barely browsed through it, having a Bible in our house was enough of religion or status of faith we would ever need. However, what good is a Bible in a home if it just collects dust while sitting on the shelf?

The Bible was meant to be opened and read by one person or many people, depending on who's in the house. Opening up the scripture allows us, the creation, to have divine fellowship with our creator. However, even though we stopped going to church, I wasn't ever done with church. I had to watch church services in the wee hours of the morning. I did that because no one was around and asleep. If I were ever caught watching church on TV, my father would have a fit. Even though I was disciplined for defying my father for watching church on TV in the later hours of the morning, I was persistent and continued to watch the services, and yes, sometimes that meant I was beaten for watching church at 10 p.m.; however, I did not care how many beatings I got, I was going to keep watching regardless.

CHAPTER 7
View From Outside the Pine Box

Scientific experts believe that a time for teenage rebellion happens between the ages of 13 and 20. I don't know if this is true; I am only going into detail about my rebellion, how deceived I was, the anger in me was never put out, and why I lost my grandmother. She struggled with heart disease for ten years, and when she passed away, I went through some dark valleys that I thought there would be no end to. On March 2, 2001. A dark cloud filled my life. One that I would be under for three years. No one had ever talked about death; it wasn't a popular subject to bring up at home or school. The end of my grandmother was something I wouldn't be ready for. I've seen many movies with big explosions and people shooting each other, but at the time, it was ok to watch because, as the viewer, you know that the scene where someone dies is only part of the script. In the end, I, as the viewer, always knew the victim/ actor would play in other movies, thus going on with his film career.

When I showed up at the funeral home, I walked into the door, and there she lay before my eyes. It destroyed me to witness that. I cried uncontrollably.

I ran up to her casket, and my mother and father held me back… I was so distraught; I was determined to get to her that I dragged my mother along with me. When I got to the front of the line, my uncles sat me down to try to be the voice of reason. He kindly explained to me, "She is gone, but think about the pain she was in for so many years. She smiled more times than anything else because you were around her; now she is at peace."

To this day, I don't think I ever really truly thanked my uncle Carmine for saying those words at the time. I say it now… Thank you. After the visitation, it was decided that my mother and father decided that I would not be going to the funeral since I reacted the way I did.

My family was too frightened that I would jump into the grave with her, so it was decided that I would miss my grandmother's funeral and burial. Perhaps the best decision my parents would ever make for me as their son. Days later, I couldn't sleep, the nightmares I had from my grandmother's passing would wear me down, and I would get insomnia for 16 months. "The pain I went through, no one will ever truly understand. I was being tortured and tormented by spiritual forces that I had no idea existed yet. Many times, I would cry myself to sleep. Many nights I asked, "God, why are you having me go through this? I need strength. I can't do this; I don't understand...." I sought day and night for answers. I would get answers to my prayer, but it would take me three years to grasp the concept of that. Because I sought answers from God, he would answer my prayers in human form. I would open the scriptures for the first time myself. Sure, I went to church as a kid, but it went in one ear and out the other as far as reading the scriptures. This time I had a purpose. I was determined to get the answers I was looking for. Tamara Norris was, at the time, my physical therapist, but as the years went on, she would become a big sister to me without even realizing it...

One day while finishing up with therapy, I told her that I had lost my grandmother and I was lost. I was a teenager in the middle of the road, and I was asked to make a decision I didn't think I was ready for. She had kindly reminded me that the Scriptures said though I walk through the valley of the shadow of death, I shall fear no evil for thou art with me. That piece of scripture stands out to me; it began to anchor me in rooted faith as the storms would come my way. The year of losing my grandmother was the most challenging thing I ever had to go through.

To make matters worse, I was going through it alone; no one in my family knew the pain I would go through daily. It hurt to breathe. Most of my family didn't even really express any amount of sadness. They just went on like it was just another day. I couldn't understand it.

Meanwhile, reading scripture was the only moments of peace I got while going through the grieving stage. It brought a sense of great peace to my soul. Even though I was watching church on TV, I still displayed anger and bitterness in my life. One of the reasons that the death of my grandmother hit me like a three-punch finishing combo is based on the fact that, even though my parents loved me, they never hugged me or even said they loved me. My grandma often went out of her way to display that to me daily to the point where it became infectious. My grandmother loved me so much that she would often risk her health and well-being just to see me bowl or play T-ball.

After my grandmother had passed away, it was like something in my family changed. Each of my family members stopped going to church; it was bizarre. I didn't understand why we went to church for ten years, and suddenly, because a family member died, church and God, in general, got put on the back burner. Yet as a teenager, I still felt it was essential to read the Bible and follow it as best as possible. Even though for many years after my grandmother's departure, I would just be spinning my wheels as far as being a real Christian was concerned. Even though I would watch faith-based programming, I would still be at war with my family on November 25, 2004. I would suffer the loss of my grandfather. In the summer of 2004, it was discovered that he had a spot of cancer on his liver.

The doctors performed surgery, and it was a success, but one week later, he contracted an infection due to the surgery. I went to see him after two weeks of being in the hospital. I walked into the room with my uncle, and his face lit up with great joy. He exclaimed to his nurses, "That's my grandson. He came to see me." Moments after arriving at the hospital, my uncle had stepped away to get coffee, and I was left in the room alone to speak and visit with my grandfather. As I was about to ask him how he was feeling, he looked into my eyes as I stood by his bedside and asked me who I was? That made me cry inside; I refused to cry in front of my grandfather when he forgot who I was. From that moment on, I knew my grandfather would not live long after that, and just a week after our visit, I got the call that my grandfather had died.

In the span of just three years, I had lost an uncle and two grandmothers, and now I was faced with the loss of my grandfather. A joke in the Italian family states that most Italians wear black because if anybody dies, *they're ready.* I didn't find that funny, I sure wasn't laughing, but I knew I was going to a lot more funerals than any typical teenager should have to. Years later, something strange happened within the inner circle. As a family, we went to the Wills of my grandparents. Although my grandparents thought of everyone regarding personal needs, it destroyed relationships between brother and sister and brother and brother. It didn't make any sense. My family was falling into chaos and arguments.

Meanwhile, I felt blessed to receive anything from the two great loves in my life. Personally, regarding how my family was acting, it was like demons were let loose in the family. It felt as if my grandparents did their best to hold them back for years, but they came to divide and destroy our family once they were passed on. It wasn't hard to see the changes within the family, but I really couldn't do anything about it because I would still battle my father for control over my life and well-being. Earlier I said that I snuck around to watch the Word of God being preached on TV. That only increased when I lost my grandparents.

I didn't want to be separated from them. I loved them so much that most of my relatives were jealous because they thought I received special attention. After all, I was different. That wasn't it; I didn't have my love at home; I was reaching out for anything…. During my trials and bouts of being oppressed, my mother was so sweet the whole time; she always came home from work and gave me the latest book by a famous preacher on the battles of the mind, knowing Jesus etc.; I believe she did this, because she may have thought and feared that I would die of a broken heart. I will tell you all the truth, the Battles of the Mind are fierce. They were so fierce that half the reason I could sleep for at least three to four hours a night was simply because of the Lord's compassion on me in hearing me weep, over and over and night after night for seven years.

While I was going through this trial, most of my family members didn't understand, and some even told me just to "get over it already." I didn't need to get over it; I needed to get Jesus. I needed his compassion to wrap me up in a shield of protection that kept me safe from all the arrows of the evil one. I needed Jesus to dry my tears and recreate my heart; I needed God that went beyond saying a hail Mary or sprinkling water on your forehead every time you entered a church.

CHAPTER 8
A Very Special Olympic History

Despite my physical limitations, I would participate in sports as a kid to be a normal boy. This period was really enjoyable for me. The only thing I found weird about the whole thing in having three siblings that were more than able to participate in sports but never did. I never understood why that was. To be born into a family where no one else but the disabled participate in sports is just weird. From ages 14 to 22, I participated in the Special Olympics. I was so competitive in sports that one sport wasn't satisfying enough. To keep up with the Jones athletically, I made a goal to participate in baseball, hockey, swimming and bowling. Still, physically I knew I could never compete in hockey because I had balance and dexterity issues. I had to find a loophole. So, I can work around my limitations without it being too much of a physical barrier for me.

That's when I found out what sledge hockey was all about. I was the tea captain of the Stratford ice breakers for four years, and you would think that as a team captain, I was very highly skilled at scoring goals; however, even though I didn't score many goals, I still have a team's record that stands today. That being spending the most time in the penalty box. Approximately I spent 9 minutes per game in the penalty box. That's five penalties. But having the lost minutes on a team for being in the penalty box makes sense, considering I was a huge wrestling fan as a teenager. When I wasn't flipping sleds over, I was competing in T ball terminates, bowling tenements and my favourite sport of all, swimming. In each sport that I competed in, I have medals and trophies.

One of the reasons I got into the Special Olympics is because my aunt wanted me to have an outlet to reduce my bound-up energy. She thought the more sorts I competed in, the happier I would be and the better home life I would have. She had a two-way thought process behind this, I'm sure raising me as a small child and a teenager was never easy on my mother; however, she knew that I couldn't participate in body-able sports. So, my aunt figured I should sign up for the Special Olympics, so my mom could get some respite, and I would have an opportunity to participate in sports at my physical level.

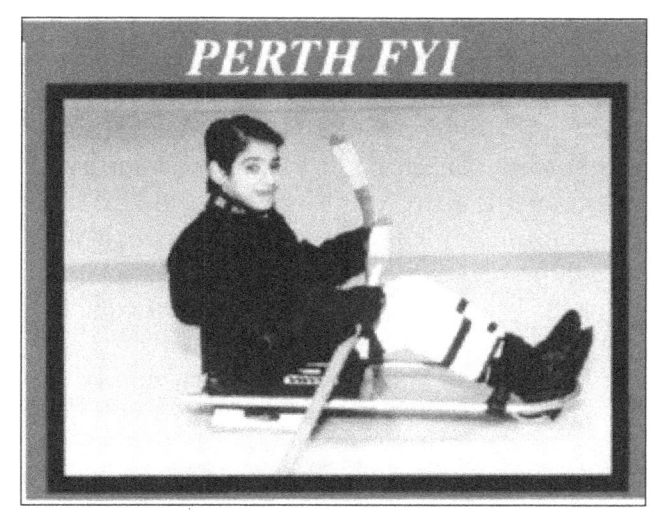

Sled Hockey Team Capitan for the Stratford Ice-Breakers March of 1999.

CHAPTER 9
Bed Pans and Bad Food

This chapter will require my readers to have a strong stomach. This is because, in the news chapter, I will be detailing my operation history. Prepare yourself, boys and girls, because each scar on my body has a story behind it. It was my parent's wish that when they first discovered I had a physical disability, they would want to correct any deformity before I knew any of it. This means I was on an operating table pretty early on in life. My first surgery took place in June of 1988. The operation was an eye surgery to correct lazy eyes. The second surgery happened in June 1992. That surgery was an operation where I got my hamstrings lengthened. The third surgery was in June of 1997. That surgery was an operation on my hamstrings. The fourth surgery was in 2007, when I was 22 years old.

    The surgeon at Victoria hospital in London decided with a team of experts that they would break both of my hips on the operating table, reposition them to the position they needed to be in, add some steel plates and a metal rod and then proceed to sew me back up. After the surgery, I was taken out of acute care after two weeks and transported to Parkwood hospital across the street, where I would perform rehab for the next four months. Therapy was good at that time, and over the next four months, I went through the paces of learning how to restrengthen every limb and re-walk. I was in therapy twice a day for an hour. Plus, I would ask physio to let me go biking in the therapy room on the weekend. My persistence would eventually pay off because when you put in two hours a day for seven days, your body will respond to that type of therapy.

    As September rolled around, I told the therapist that you have to train myself to walk without a walker in August. I have to go to college, and I need to have endurance if I'm going to last in college. They agreed to put any extra time to help me by having me walk with a walker around a pavilion, hopping on one foot and then asking me to switch the feet when I came back around the other pavilion. Their method of madness hurt like hell, but it worked. On September 7, 2007, I enrolled in college for the first time, and the only reason I was able to do that was that I had a good physical therapist at the rehab centre. Keep in mind that when I left Parkwood in 2007, the therapist said my body was strong enough that I didn't need a walker anymore. So, throughout my five years in college, I did not use a walker once.

CHAPTER 10
A Protein Shake and A Weight Room

Before I begin this chapter, I want to preface this chapter by letting my readers know that I suffered from my father as a small little Anthony, greatly from a severe eating disorder brought on by the home life that I went through. My mother didn't think I would make it past ten years old, and when I did, she expected me to die at 12 or 13. But even though I didn't die, I was hospitalized several times for malnourishment. Here are the facts about that period...

Now, as a person with cerebral palsy who could walk and talk like any other boy, the only problem with that is that because of my disability and the amount of energy I would use up to move, it would often leave 10-year-old me worn out and exhausted every single day I went to school. At first, my parents thought wearing myself out at the end of the day was great, but after a few months and a keen eye, my mother looked at how thin I was after looking at my rib cage.

My mom quickly realized that I would have to go through some health changes with the amount of energy that my body would use. The only problem with that is that my parents didn't know where to look at first. Well, it's a good thing as a youngster, I needed a computer to write complete sentences. My mother did much looking around, and she discovered through networking and reaching out to people that I could use a respite worker. This worker would help me do physiotherapy and take me to the gym, allowing me to experience life outside my jail cell of a home.

I say that my home was similar to a jail cell because the relationship I would share with the male counterpart with my mother was a very, very, very abusive one, and that's putting it mildly.

Anytime I would go to the table to eat any food, Emperor Nero would be right there with his hand squeezing the back of my neck and in the other hand would be my spoon. He would pick it up and shove the spoon down my throat to the point where I would taste the spoon's metal. During a doctor's appointment, I went to see a nutritionist; I had seen him many times before. However, at age 13, this appointment was a little different. At first, the doctor did the usual checkup—weight, bone test, and a skin colour test. However, after the usual checkup was finished, he asked my father to wait outside while I went to talk with the doctor inside a private room.

The doctor was very open and upfront with me; he began to say, "Anthony, you are very sick and unwell." You are severely underweight, and you could die." Is that what you want?" I responded, Absolutely Not! I don't have an eating disorder, but I do have much stress at suppertime; I began to tell the doctor that every time I eat at my house, it's like World War 3. I often get abused even before I can pick up my spoon. The doctor then followed up my response by asking the million-dollar question. The doctor asked me was, what will it take you to eat? I answered... My response to the question was that I have no problem eating at other people's homes; there are various people that I visit, and often I eat at their houses with no problem whatsoever, and their questions were all the same. "Anthony, how come you eat at other houses, and you don't eat at your own. My response was because you don't have your hands around my neck, screaming, eat you, lousy kid."

The doctor looked at me with shock and awe.

He said, okay, I think I have the whole story. He then asked me to leave the room so he could talk to my father in private. I agreed and left the room. The doctor sat my father down and asked him the same questions that earlier I had answered to see if the stories were true and matched up with what I was saying. Being the type of person he was, Nero wouldn't waste time in admitting that he was using physical and verbal abuse so that I may eat. According to the emperor's understanding, "he was doing that for my benefit to keep me alive." The doctor told my father, "Perhaps you need to stop being so forceful with him; you're damaging the boy." My father stormed out of the office screaming, no one will tell me how to raise my son." As we drove home that day, Nero began to curse at me for the entirety of the 45-minute drive back to our house.

After hearing all the cursing, I had to endure; I decided to punish my parents by going on a hunger strike for four days.

In those four days, I did not talk to a single person; I just stayed in my room and survived on water from the bathroom faucet.

After four days, I emerged from my room, all smiles... Even though my parents were shocked that I was still alive, my father Nero was furious that I was smiling and hadn't eaten in four days. I guess he expected me to beg him for food, but I wouldn't give him the satisfaction. I knew going through a hunger strike may have seemed a little much, but I felt like, at the time, I needed to prove a point of who is stronger. As a kid, I claimed it was a battle of endurance and a battle of wits, but in reality, it was all about sorrow and ego. I wanted to hurt my family by proving that I don't need them because real families show love to each other; they are not abusive.

To give the readers a glimpse of life from ages 6-14. I was approximately 40 pounds soaking wet for the next seven years. It wasn't until I went into the eighth grade that I started gaining weight, and that was only because I was on a protein shake that I drank three times a day. After a month of being on the protein shake and weight gainer, I would gain 30 pounds in three months. When I started gaining weight and began feeling better, I began working out because I had a new lease on life; now I know what you're thinking... "You grew up a wrestling fan, so did you train like Hulk Hogan by taking your vitamins? The answer is no. Every time I picked a pair of weights or did a squat with my trainers, it didn't take me too long to realize that my main focus during working out should be endurance and conditioning because, as a physically disabled person, I often treated my body like that of a multi-sport professional athlete.

CHAPTER 11
The Pen is Mightier than the Sword – The Journalism Years

So there I was, at 23 years old. My future was set in stone, or so I thought. I would go to college to study journalism. At first thought, I didn't know what to think, but I thought about the quest more. The more I became confident in my ability; I was a natural-born storyteller and writer. I just needed the skills to become good. I had the aspiration but not the skill. I accepted Ms. Mohr's offer, and I was well on my way to starting college; because it was my first year in a big city, the only option was to move into a college residence. I quietly thought, "What have I done? What did I get myself into?" To most first years, their first year of college would seem like a dream because of the sense of freedom that most students would feel they rightly deserved. However, my first year of college felt like a nightmare that I couldn't wake up from.

Everywhere I turned, students were getting drunk and on drugs. I couldn't believe it; I had culture shock. As the year progressed, I realized that studying journalism wasn't fun. I had many more reports and assignments than my brain and hands could manage. A typical day in college starts at eight o'clock in the morning and finishes class at six o'clock in the evening. The more I thought about it, the more I realized quickly that I had no life. I studied all day in school, and when I got home, I would sleep for the next five hours after coming home from school only to study again. I put my body through so much unnecessary physical and mental strain. To study six to seven classes a semester was starting to catch up with me. I didn't like it. I was facing burnout. The only reason I survived the semester is that I had the joy of coming home on weekends. At home, I would catch up on all my missed sleep.

I could only run the race for so long before I would collapse. To my professors, the stresses the students were facing were normal. Another reason I didn't like to study journalism was that we had to research so much depressing news. It warped my mind. After the school year ended, I came home to sleep for the next few months, in April of 2009. I watched WrestleMania 25 live from Houston. I paid close attention to one match; in particular, it was a match featuring two athletes who were often named the best in the business. Shawn Michaels and The Undertaker, I was blown away and captivated by the action. I decided to break into the wrestling business.

When I returned to school, I had the mindset that I would use my journalism degree to work for the WWE one day. The only problem was that I was not the best in the new writing class. I didn't watch the news that often, and frankly, not paying attention to the news hurt me. I paid the price by failing the class. So for me, in the summer of 2009, the question became, how would I pass journalism if I hated the news. The answer to that question is a complex one indeed. The short answer is I had wrestler, rockstar and New York Times bestselling author teach me summer school. In college, students are given four months off. Most students use this time away from the classroom to go to work to save money for their next year of college tuition. I, however, had different things in mind. In the summer of 2009, I walked into my local Chapters and picked up what would be my very first wrestling biography. I first bought the wrestling titled, *A Lion's Tale, Around the World in Spandex,* written by Chris Jericho.

CHAPTER 12
Climbing Mount Olympus Without Leaving My Backyard

As much as I want to put Mr. Jericho over as the greatest writer of all time, right next to Roald Dahl, R. L. Stine and Mark Twain, I have to admit I did have other influences in my life that allowed me to be successful when it came to returning inside the journalism classroom. Although his first written book encouraged me to go to journalism school, understanding the different print styles goes back to ancient Greece.

In the Spring of 2008 and 2009, I was given an ultimatum before the summer break in May. As I said earlier in the book, I didn't know the type of writing style that I needed to be successful in the program enough to have passing grades. When I went into the Chair of Journalism's office, the two professors sat me down and closed the door behind them. Mark, the program chair, said, "Anthony, we have called for you to come here today because your news writing teacher and I are very concerned about your grades, and we want to figure out why they are low." When they said and gestured that my grades were low, my journalism grades were 38-45% average. Way below the class average of 78%.

After discussing the matter with me for a few brief moments, they decided that they wanted to dismiss me from the program. I pleaded with them not to make that decision; I explained to them that in my early school years, I wasn't given the proper time frame to work on assignments and sometimes, in school, rather than the teachers explain the mistakes, they would decide to pass me. This method being used early on in my education would lead to years of me trying to play catch up with the rest of the students. I pleaded with the professors again to change their minds because I had a passion for writing, I just told them that I needed to learn the mechanics of it and I could become a better writer. They agreed to give me another shot, and I knew after the meeting was over that I had to prove to them that this journalism program was for me.

During the summer months away from Conestoga College, I spent my time in chapters. I was buying up wrestling books and novels of Greek Mythology. Why did I choose to learn about Greek Mythology? In truth, I thought there was a correlation between the mythical hero Hercules and the pro wrestling world. However, I did face various challenges. For instance, during my time in journalism, I didn't make it a well-known secret that I was a wrestling fan to anybody that would listen. My professors didn't like me being a wrestling fan because, in their mind, I would use my experiences inside this prestigious college to work for the WWE and do Broadcasting for a pseudo sport? I was blinded by fame and bright lights in my professor Larry's... Larry always assumed that one of his journalism students working for a well-known worldwide wrestling corporation was laughable. More on that story a little while later...

Let's take you, the readers, back to my summer of buying books at Chapters. I knew that I would have any success in the fall in news writing; I had to bear down and read a book front to back. I wasn't much of a book reader. It wasn't that I couldn't read; I actually could read very well. However, I found that reading a book that didn't have anything to do with sports is boring .... I was a sports guy through and through. At the beginning of May, I wanted to answer a question I had asked myself. What are the origins of the English language? Ancient Greek, of course. As a child, I knew about the story of Hercules from the long-running TV series featuring Kevin Sorbo, not Ryan Gossling, but I found books by Homer rather complex and confusing.

I wanted to read a book with plenty of action without all the poetry and hidden innuendos. So, as I was walking down every aisle, waiting for a book to jump out at me, I came across Percy Jackson and the *Lightning Thief,* a book series by Rick Riordan. The book covers looked awesome, so I decided to buy the series as a whole... I read the entire five books in three months, but I did so by reading out loud... I read the books aloud to begin to understand how the words sound coming off the page at me. I thought maybe that might help me in the classroom when I return in the fall...

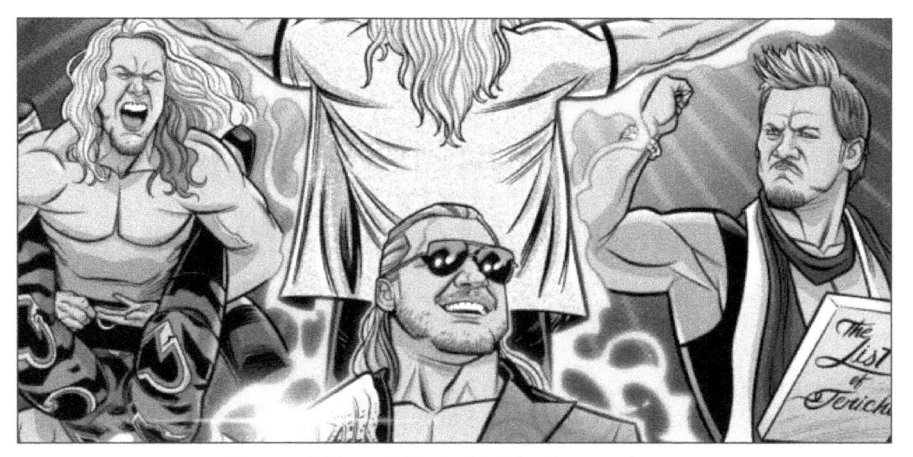

The evolution of Chris Jericho in a cartoon.

I enjoyed reading the book series, and when I found out that Percy Jackson the *Lightning Thief and Sea of Monsters* was going to be turned into a movie, I was excited. Still, after watching the two films, I realized the director only got one thing right... That's the casting of Annabeth Chase, portrayed by Alexandra Daddario... (Excuse me for a moment while I raise an eyebrow.) So, after reading the entire book series, I went back to school in the fall. I sat in my chair listening to the news writing professor speak, and after completing an assignment, I was given a 65% the first week back, then the following week for the next project; I got a 71% and then an 81%.

After about a month, Larry pulled me aside and said, "Anthony, I am impressed with your new writing assignments. What did you do differently from the previous semester?"

I told him, "Nothing really; I just studied Greek Mythology books and read the books aloud to understand writing tones, and the best part is, I didn't have to leave my backyard." I will never forget the importance of reading out loud. I will never forget the sense of accomplishment I felt when I got my term report card. My grades for the class were completely different. I went from a student with a 38-45% average to a student with an average of 74%.

When my professor looked at me as I reviewed my term grades, he said, "Good job Anthony," that was worth more than graduating with ten college diplomas.

CHAPTER 13

Caught Between the Ropes Chasing a Lion's Tale, The Ray Barone Life

They say sometimes life imitates art. In my case, that was true. At 23, when I went to college, my father wanted me to pick a career that would change the world. There was only one issue I had with that set of ideals. I didn't think there was a career made for me. After all, only the cool kids got to pick the real awesome jobs. Careers like being a police officer, a firefighter or a soldier in the military. I knew I was never going to qualify for all the career choices. The only thing I was remotely interested in was sports and writing. So, one day in the summer of 2006, I commented to my brother Angelo after watching the television show *Everybody Loves Raymond*, "I would love to work in sports." As it would turn out, my brother Angelo wanted to go to college to become a police officer. As I said, life imitates art...

When my brother and the rest of the family got word that I wanted to go to college to be a sports writer, they scoffed and said, "he's going to want to become a professional wrestler. I know how his mind works, said Mom." However, I knew there was no way I could even attempt something like that in the back of my mind. I liked wrestling. That much is true, but to say I had dreams of becoming like a John Cena-type character is misunderstood. I wanted to become a sportswriter for the wrestling industry. Now I am not the person to put too much stake in fate. However, when you're watching TSN and SPORTSNET every day just for the highlights, even though you have already seen the game live. Perhaps the world is trying to tell you something... After reading more wrestling biographies, like *Hardcore Diaries*, by Mick Foley, books by Ted Dibiase, Dave Bautista and others, it didn't take me long to decide which sport I wanted to get involved in. I had to ask myself one question: would I get involved in professional wrestling? I did what any tech-savvy 20-something-year-old would do. I asked Google. More specifically, I looked around for websites that would pay me to write articles for me just to watch wrestling. It worked within two weeks. I had two part-time jobs as a wrestling writer, and I went to school full time.

I was living the college dream. I worked for a few companies called ring rap.com and Rant Sports.com. I enjoyed it, but after a little while, I wanted more articles. I did yet another Google search, and I ran across the name of Greg Oliver (a Canadian wrestling journalist and author. He was the editor of the Slam Sports wrestling division. My responsibilities included calling up whatever wrestler I was asked to set a time for an interview either by phone or email. Then after the game of 21 questions was over, I would sift through the nonsense and write the articles.

When my time with Slam Sports compromised my days in the journalism classroom, I chose to look for a company I could work for that would allow me never to miss class again but still keep my passion for writing and wrestling intact. I worked part-time at indie shows doing colour commentary in my quest to become a wrestling journalist jack of all trades. To multi-task and gain experience, I applied to work for a small independent wrestling show as a colour commentator at Kitchener's Tri-City Wrestling. After a few months at TCW, I was asked to have a chat with one of the wrestlers.

"I have been watching you on commentary, and you come alive."

I laughed, saying, "It's just Chris Jericho with the volume turned up to 15."

"I heard you're studying journalism at Conestoga College," he said, and I nodded in agreement.

"I have a friend that wants to start a women's wrestling magazine, and he needs a lead editor," he added.

Working as head editor at *Ring Sirens* magazine was pretty cool. I got to see the women's evolution of wrestling long before it ever came on WWE television. I was the magazine's top editor in a year, writing four to five stories a month. My interviews also made the cover of seven of 12 issues.

In 2012, I was an accomplished website wrestling writer: a magazine writer and a local independent wrestling commentator. I was the Cameron Crowe of independent wrestling. After a year, though, it became too expensive to run a magazine, so the company closed down, and I sought out the American Dream...

I wanted to make a splash south of the border because I wanted to start my career before I became 30 years old. So, I had the idea of submitting some work to Pro Wrestling Illustrated with Stu Sacks. I waited to hear back from PWI before the two weeks were up. God intervened that would change my direction in life altogether. During my waiting period on Pro Wrestling Illustrated, there was one night I developed Carbon Monoxide Poisoning. After being taken to local emerge after collapsing and being found by a friend of mine as I was sprawled out on the floor, the doctors on call determined that I had co2 and that it was fortunate that I made it to emerge before I died. After that life-changing experience, I wanted to change direction in my life before it fell apart.

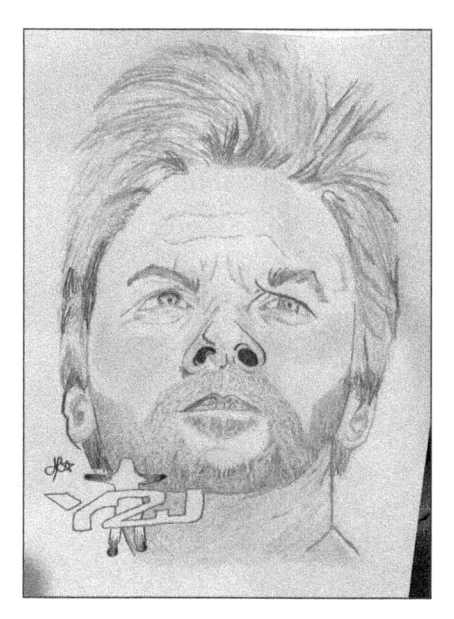

**A sketch of Chris Jericho as a wrestling bad guy.
Artist Alyssa Perriera.**

CHAPTER 14

There is ACTION in Akron

A baptism by fire is a lot different than a baptism by water. To understand the difference, I've written this chapter. Churchgoing Christians believe that baptism by water is a statement made by human beings to live a life for God. It is true. However, baptism by water is clearly only always for a clear conscience. To live a life for God means to live holy, and there's more to living holy than just a confession of sin. To live holy means you have to abstain from sins. To live holy lives up to live free from all sin. That's why in the sermon on the mount, Jesus had been therefore holy, even as your Father in heaven which is holy. Matthew : King James Version (KJV)

> [48] Be ye therefore perfect, even as your Father which is in heaven is perfect.

When it comes to getting baptized by water the Scriptures recognize the difference so why can't the human race me as understand that action means in a different result. Matthew 3:11, King James Version (KJV)

> [11] I indeed baptize you with water unto repentance. but he that cometh after me is mightier than I, whose shoes I am not worthy to bear: he shall baptize you with the Holy Ghost, and with fire:

I thought I was good enough to get into heaven for many years because I didn't kill or bring harm to anybody. I had different sins that I dealt with. And through a series of circumstances, I would come to know that I would either be freed from all sin or be captive to my sin and die in them. I realized quickly that a form of godliness like going to church wasn't what the Christian life was truly about. About two months after my baptism, before I knew it, the world became a product of my environment. Before I knew it, I became lukewarm. Accepted the word of man and not God's. This was because I wanted to change the world and everything in it. The more I chased the world more trouble I got into. A life of sexual morality was at my doorstep. However, it didn't take me long to realize that I was wrong in giving over to the flesh. I am 29 years old, and if there's anything in life that I could take back, it would be my virginity. However, I can't take that back; what happened then happened in the past, and now I have a life washed in the blood of Jesus. The same blood that washed away all my sins. Now I live to speak to others without why having one's virginity until their wedding night is so important. Suppose a man not keep his virginity. He is likely to be a captive of his flesh without realizing it. How did I come is this knowledge? I got baptized by fire.

I went to the upper room and tarried for seven days until I received the gift of speaking in tongue as the spirit gave them utterance. One night, I came into this knowledge while watching a good friend of mine praying. At that time, I was seeking God but was unsure if I was ready because I didn't know if I was worthy, and for that matter, I also didn't know if I was clean enough to be a vessel of the Holy Ghost. That night I prayed with my friends Scott, Tamara and their three kids, Jacob, Jamie and Jenna. As I looked over at Scott, I heard some Hebrew come out of his mouth. I was on my knees, and I suddenly looked over to listen to him better, and he was speaking so fast, I couldn't understand what was happening. I was speechless. Imagine that the boy who loves to talk was finally silent.

The more I prayed through to God; my tongue started to twirl tangle up words. Faster and faster, I stammered for 25 minutes. I continued to pray earnestly because I saw evidence of the Holy Ghost even though I didn't know what was happening at the time as soon as I saw Scott receive a new tongue. I said to myself, okay, I guess this is real…. The day after I went back to school, the school didn't seem the same to me.

I was more aware of the differences between evil and good. I came into the reality of the two factions. Seven days later, while praying again, I received the baptism by fire, and because I received the new experience, I came out of the world. I didn't want anything in the world. The only thing that was outside my grasp was the truth and knowledge about God. I began to change the way I dressed, spoke, and acted. I began to change what I listened to. I became very cautious about what I will watch and read. I felt free, but I also felt burdened. I felt free from all sin, but I felt burdened because I wanted to do what was right could do to speak to people about God, thus saving them from the torture of tribulation.

When I received the baptism by fire, my church friends didn't know what had happened to me. They called me to come back to church. I refused to. I received the baptism of the Holy Ghost; I became a man. I became a man with a passion for the lost; I became a man who wanted to win souls for God at any cost to become a man who always wanted to stand on a solid rock foundation. I became a man that always wanted to study to show myself prove rightly dividing the word of God. I became a man that wanted to walk hand-in-hand with God.

I became a man who wanted to prove himself worthy in the eyes of God. I became a man who wanted to study his word so much that I wanted to become familiar with that I do my own hands and feet. For foundations like wrestling, women, studying world history and even reading about Greek mythology put me in danger of sinking into the sand. Paul said it best in his letter to the Corinthian church that when I was a child, I reasoned like a child; I thought like a child, but when I became a man, put away childish things. In reality and honesty, everything before God that I ever did I count now as dung.

CHAPTER 15
Going to Bible College on a Greyhound

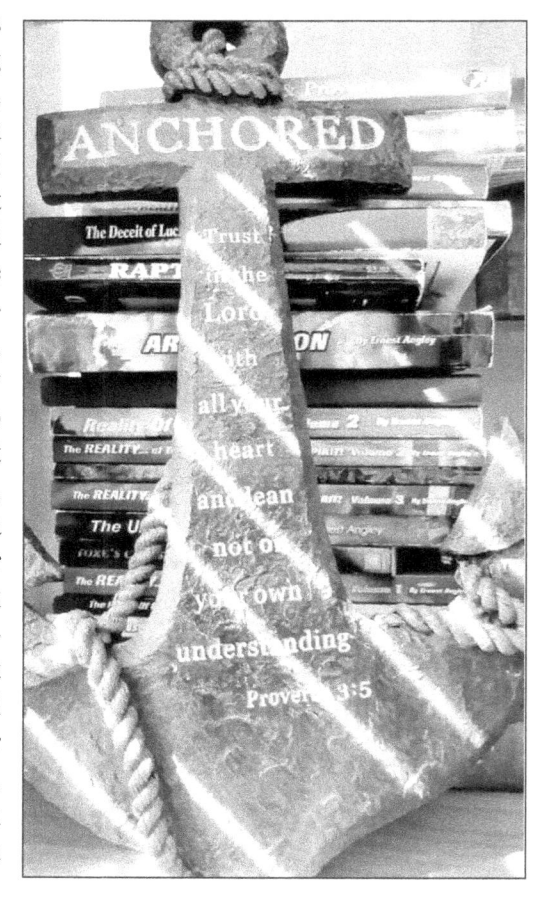

When God woke me up from my slumber, and I wasn't too eager to jump back into the sports world right away, I wanted to look for a job that would allow me to use my journalism talents. In 2019, I was at a weird time in my life. My life goals had just changed, and I needed to find a job where I could use my writing and verbal talents. I thought about it for a bit. As confident as I was about wanting another job, but this time, my focus had to be on working for the Lord; I was still unsure about what I wanted to do and how I could work for the Lord. I didn't know anything until August 20, 2020. That was the day my twin brother Angelo asked me to be his best man on his wedding date, September 20, 2020. As a whole, my twin brother was always going to pick me as his best man. Although he made me sweat it out after a day and said it's either you or another guy. I simply asked him, "Angelo, I don't think Corey ever shared a womb with you; make the right decision." When he agreed to have me as his best man, I went right to work.

I was only given two rules for instructions which I entirely ignored, by the way. My mother had said, please don't say anything that is embarrassing for us. My brother also added that I must not add in any biblical scripture. However, as I said, I completely ignored those two rules. I made concessions of my own. "I kindly told my mother and my brother that the best man speech will be written the way I choose, and if I need to add scripture into the speech, then it will be added. I refused to compromise on this issue. I didn't want to stray away from the truth and be censored for the sake of convenience."

After two weeks of writing the best man speech, it was complete. The speech itself wasn't going to send anybody to the depths of Hades.

The Best Man Wedding Speech

How Can You Measure a Heart?

Even though we may be twins the circumstances behind our birth did not determine the wedding party order. As I sat down to write a heartfelt speech, my mind began to wander; there I sat, a feathered ink pen in one hand and a piece of papyrus paper in front of me and beside me, a candle illuminating the words of the pages of the scroll. As I began to write, some of the world's greatest writers in literature ran through my mind. Names that were my childhood heroes as I grew up. Those names include Robert Munsch, R.L. Stine, Dr. Seuss and Roald Dahl. As I woke up daydreaming, I realized I don't have Goosebumps and pigs belong between two hot dog buns and not between the pages of a children's book. That being said, I considered being my brother's best man on his wedding day my Golden ticket.

I often get asked how do you and your brother get along so well? The answer is simple, when it comes to video games you will never be without a player two. When it comes to video games Angelo is the Mario to my Luigi but today, he changed the game because he got himself a Princess Peach. At age 23, my brother and I decided to part ways and went to separate schools. Angelo received an acceptance letter to attend Fanshawe College in London to study Police Foundation. While I received a high letter of recommendation to attend Conestoga College to study journalism. The Robert and Ray Barone dream was becoming a reality. A year into my studies, my brother informed me that he no longer wanted to become a policeman but rather a protector of wildlife. I kindly remind my brother Angelo just what my father does for a winter recreational activity, and I asked him if he was sure about wanting to become a game warden for conservation areas. I also took the time to remind my twin brother that the camouflage my father wears in the wintertime during dear and moose season isn't because he is trying to make a fashion statement. Wedding traditions are status quo such as the married couple would eat a piece of the wedding cake on the eve, they're of the first anniversary but as you may expect Italian traditions work a bit differently. As Europeans, our lives are centered around cultural ideals. such as food and a strong method of communication known as yelling or fussing. I stated earlier Italian's love to make food. We love to make enough food to feed an army. An Italian dinner looks like a huge math problem that would stunt most sports banquets. Here's how the numbers break down, add 10 to 12 chairs depending on the company and multiply the food portions depending on the mouths to feed. If my calculations are correct, you have a table size 28 feet long, which makes sense why Italians are always yelling at each other because they're always yelling at each other to pass the food around the table. It's time for Angelo and Jessie to start a relationship that does not include yelling or fussing. They can do that by putting love at the centre of their marriage. What is love? Webster's dictionary defines love as a strong sense of companionship with another person. However, each year, the definition of love changes according to romance novels, dictionaries and even federal laws. I have a few words for the parents to mark this occasion.

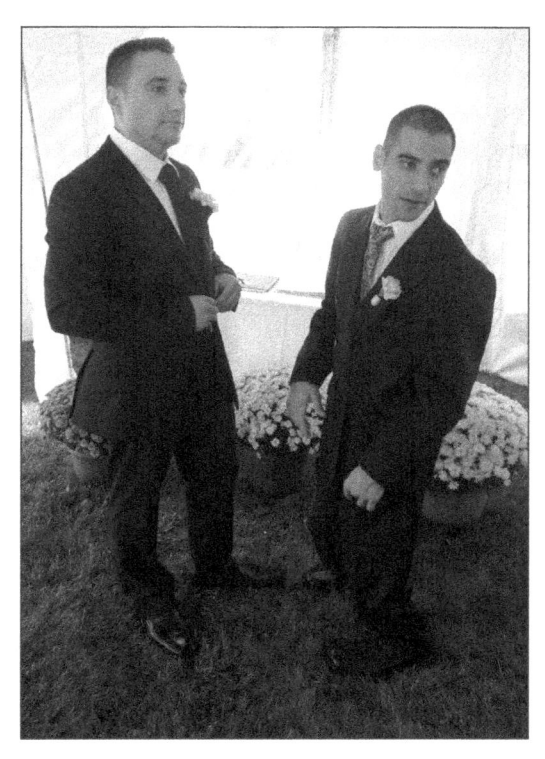

Taking a photo with Angelo as his best man on his wedding day, September 2015.

The Book of Mark, chapter 10, verse 16: "Behold I send you amongst the wolves as sheep be as harmless as doves but as wise as serpents." These two people have become one flesh in the sight of God and all of us. It is written in the Scriptures that a man must leave his mother and father and holdfast to his wife. As the bride and groom both rise, I would like to remind them that my definition of love kindly isn't coming from a worldly standpoint. My definition of love is best found in the Scriptures in first Corinthians chapter 13.

> Love does not give up. Love is kind. Love is not jealous. Love does not put itself up as being important. Love has no pride. Love does not do the wrong thing. Love never thinks of itself. Love does not get angry. Love does not remember the suffering of being

hurt by someone. Love is not happy with sin. Love is satisfied with the truth. Love takes everything that comes without giving up. Love believes all things. Love hopes for all things. Love keeps on in all things. When I was a child, I spoke like a child. I thought like a child. I understood like a child. Now I am a man. I do not act like a child anymore. And now we have these three: faith and hope and love, but the greatest of these is love. May the Lord bless you both in this marriage...

After my brother's wedding was over, I went home, and I quickly realized after receiving a ten-minute standing ovation that I was encouraged that God could use me in a good way.

Later on, I was told that God would be very proud of my work for him, maybe helping produce books... I thought that was a great idea, but Reverend Ernest Angley also asked me that I should take the online Bible College. I did because I thought if I went to the Bible College, I could always get a job preaching alongside the three ministers. I thought taking the Bible college classes online was a great idea because if the church needed an extra hand, I would be more than willing to fill in... If ever I was called to preach, then I would never be out of a job because everyone either gets married or buried.

I enjoyed taking the Online Bible College. I eventually got certified in the span of four years. I even improved my average in theology studies of 91% when taking my final exams. I liked going to Ohio via Greyhound; even though the travel was long in the beginning, I was happy I was going to take more lessons through the Bible College, and I was pleased that whenever I had to start a new branch of courses, I would travel to Ohio to get more material. I know what you may be thinking. "Wait, you took a Greyhound bus to Ohio to go to church and pick up extra class materials? The answer is yes, and yes, there is a reason I did this. The reason behind why is simple. If I wanted a pair of Mickey Mouse ears, do I order them from Amazon, or if I have the opportunity to go to Disneyland, do I go to Disneyland myself and enjoy the whole experience...

CHAPTER 16
Help, A Hard Thing For a Man to Ask

In the fall of 2018, after I had completed Bible College, I decided it was time to get an apartment of my own. All my life I spent living with people. In the summer, I went on the lookout for an apartment, and although I didn't get all the things I wanted with the apartment, I did get a more than a fair price, plus the place was open concept. However, I knew that I would live on my own for the first time. I needed some help. I went through various agencies that would help with anything from showering, shaving, dressing, and cooking... These agencies that helped me out at home were more than excellent, but in October of 2018, I began to become very ill and very tired.

After being extremely tired for about two, I finally got an appointment to see my family doctor. The doctor believed at the time that I was suffering from a sinus infection. As two more weeks passed, I booked another appointment to see the doctor this time; I explained to him that I was extremely unwell directly after I ate. After answering some questions, he determined that I had an ulcer, but he wanted to be sure. After an endoscopy exam, I discovered that I didn't just have one ulcer, but four ulcers were located on my esophagus, two on each side.

In addition to the complicated medical issues I was having inside my throat, the doctor would also tell me that I had severe damage to my throat. Still, there was nothing he could have done because he was not a specialist in gastro issues. To make matters worse, even though I was put on medication to alleviate some of the problems, the ulcers were too far advanced in my throat for the medication to be as effective. A few months after I found out I had ulcers, another medical issue came up. One night while sleeping, I turned on my left side and, in the morning, I couldn't move my legs. The morning I woke, my legs and feet felt like cinder blocks.

I couldn't believe it. My first thought was, "Anthony, what happened to you? Move your feet." But I couldn't. Immediately after about five minutes, I tried to roll, and I let out a terrifying monster-like scream.

The only saving grace during these moments of shock was that I had Cerebral Palsy; I had a social worker connect me with an agency called the Victoria Order of Nurses. Or the VON for short. I had my phone beside my bed, and I made two phone calls; the first phone call was to my doctor. I explained to her that I couldn't move my legs, to which she said. "I will pencil you in right away. Get here at 11 am. I said OKAY," and then I hung up the phone to call my nursing aides to help me get showered and dressed.

The time was 8:30 am, and I don't even remember taking time to have breakfast that morning before my appointment because I was worried that I might have pinched a nerve and paralyzed myself. I hated to think of such things, but when you can't move your legs, and you don't have answers yet, your mind goes. I had great fear that I did indeed become partially paralyzed, and that thought scared me half to death. Part of the reason I feared becoming paralyzed was that I remember reading the story of the mother of Chris Jericho becoming paralyzed in an accident.

When I first read about the accident, I was 24 years old, and it took a lot for me to break down, but I did because, for the majority of my life, I heard all the naysayers scoff and say to me that I would be in a wheelchair when I am 30 years old. The story of her accident and paralysis would force me to work around my physical barriers so I wouldn't end up in a wheelchair. When I began working out, my focus was not to become The Hulk but rather on strength, stamina and conditioning. I failed to see the big picture as BIG of a wrestling fan as I was. I could not know that I was in a wrestling match, and I had been in one my entire life. My opponent was my body. By staying in top physical shape, I was five steps ahead of the disability. However, when I couldn't feel my legs the morning I woke up, I will admit, cerebral palsy put me in a sleeper hold. I say this honestly because, after all the X-rays of my bones and CT scans of my stomach, it became a waiting period for me. I hated waiting for things to happen, considering I was so sick, but I couldn't do anything; I had to remain patient. When you as an individual are dealing with multiple health issues, being patient isn't your top priority.

In the chapter, I remember that even though I had moved out on my own, I didn't get everything I had wanted, but I was okay because the price was right for the time. Well, I had to sacrifice one of my perks. I was told to live with roommates. I was okay with that even though my roommates at the time had a sexual appetite like Pitbull's chewing on a steak. Keep in mind; that I had just finished Bible College, so I kept my nose clean and out of trouble. When my housemates weren't putting notches in their bedposts, they were somewhat nice guys. However, hormones and alcohol can be a dangerous mix. Nevertheless, I would endure through this time. In February 2019, something strange began to happen with the world; people started getting randomly sick worldwide, and some were even dying of a virus known as the Coronavirus or COVID-19. In March of 2019, COVID-19 outbreaks became an everyday occurrence. The virus became so bad worldwide that even the World Health Organization called it a global crisis.

Day by day, it wasn't uncommon for you to hear that in one single day, 1,500 to 3,000 died every day all around the world and as the virus spread, the numbers began to rise higher. As the number of deaths increased, the domino effect worldwide is still something felt even today. Countries around the world started wearing face masks and protective shields. Businesses were affected as the government stepped in to stop the spread of the virus by limiting people going to stores. Due to the outbreak worldwide, every facet of life was controlled by the government. Wedding attendance, Funeral gatherings, bars and restaurants were closed. From elementary to university, schools on every level were all closed down. If people refused to obey the government's rules, fines were handed down.

Due to the effects of COVID-19, my roommates who were attending university had classes cancelled. I panicked personally because I thought if my roommates weren't going to school, they would go to the bar every night and bring home their "drunken prize." However, as St Patrick's Day approached, there was a massive shutdown. After the shutdown of all restaurants, various people left the apartment building to go home and be with their families. With 80% of the building gone home because of the global pandemic, I was left alone to live by myself. I have to be honest because I was the only one of my roommates to stay in the apartment; I felt like I had just won an episode of survivor... Perhaps though, it was best that I didn't have anybody living with me at the time because my health issues only became worse. It became such a challenge for my pride to ask for help from people to shower me and dress me because I was so weak.

CHAPTER 17
Ulcers and Ambulance Rides

It was undoubtedly the worst time that I had ever experienced during this period when I say my sickness with ulcers became increasingly worse. I am not sugar coding anything. I got to the point where I put my VON workers through a disastrous environment. Many of them took care of me and cleaned up vomit three times a day. I often felt terrible for them because I didn't mean to toss my cookies everywhere about the apartment. The vomiting constantly became so bad that I would go on to ruin blankets, clothes, mattresses, and even the floors and walls of my bedroom were covered in puke. It was a terrible time.

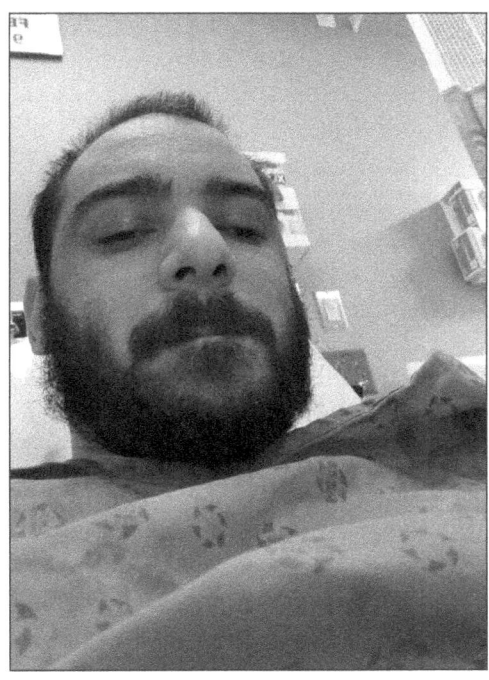

First Hospital visit with bleeding ulcers May 4, 2019.

I remember the first time I ended up bleeding after vomiting because I was new to what to look for; I just sat there dizzy after throwing up one day around 5 p.m. and experiencing dizziness. I decided to call the Healthline on-call nurse. I kindly told her, "I don't know what to do; I am very dizzy and have a history of cerebral palsy, but I have never felt like this before with my disability." She asked me if I had any other medical conditions; I told her yes, I do. I let her know that I currently have ulcers in my esophagus. She then asked me if I had thrown up at all that day and what was the colour of the bile? I told her it was dark... Without another question, she hastily demanded that I go to the nearest hospital right away because you have internal bleeding.

She said you need to get to the hospital as soon as possible." When I hung up the phone with the nurse, I called the taxi to take me to the hospital...

When I arrived at Victoria Hospital, I was immediately given a blood test and asked by the nurse to wait to speak with the on-call doctor. Four and half hours later, the doctor walks in and says, *"You have lost quite a bit of blood, Anthony; we have to keep you with us for a while. I said, okay. I will stay for a few hours while this gets under control."* The doctor dismissed that comment and said, "You don't understand; your blood is deficient. I don't want you to go home like this; if you do without proper treatment, you will fall asleep and won't wake up." After the doctor said that, the next question I asked before rolling up my sleeves so that they could quickly get an IV in me was, "what is my blood count and what is considered a low number?" He answered, "your blood count is 78. Normally it is supposed to be 130-160..."

The next day I contacted my cousin in Italy and told him what had happened. Within 30 minutes, my uncle from Italy had called me to comfort me during a time of great stress. He simply told me not to be afraid and let the doctors help me. I agreed with him, and the next day I had an endoscopy in my room. After five days of IV, my blood count went up to 100. Because of this, the hospital decided to release me, figuring that my numbers would only increase, but for the next two weeks, I was so tired that I made a call to the doctor.

When I got to see the doctor, she wanted to do a blood test, and then I went home. A few days later, the doctor's office called to give me the results. The nurse on the phone told me that my blood count was 106. She went on to say, the doctor would like to put you on iron pills. Over the next little while, I started to feel less dizzy and tired. However, I kept bursting open, so I was rushed to the hospital several times in three months. The next visit to emerge. The on-call doctors told me that I had developed a hiatal hernia. I asked the doctors in the hospital what do I do about it. They said, "we can't do anything about it." They would go on to give me more medications and send me home... After visiting the emerge several more times for puking dark bile and being released shortly after. I would ask for a local dietitian to visit me. On the morning she visited me, I threw up in front of her. So, she signed some special paperwork so I could go on a government-assisted diet for people with severe weight loss. After getting sick in front of her, she said, "you seem to be struggling with your stomach. I hope you get it fixed sometime soon."

After she left, I began to research the information behind hiatal hernia a short time later. I eventually found out that there was a type of surgery to help me with what I was going through. I even watched the surgeries being performed on other patients, thanks to YouTube. After a few months of research, my family doctor got me to have an appointment with a thoracic surgeon. The date was January 17, 2021. I met the doctor and signed papers to have the surgery done in three months' time. I, of course, had to wait three months because the world was in the middle of a global health crisis with COVID-19. The surgery for my hernia repair was scheduled for late March to mid-February. However, just one week later, my body decided it couldn't wait. On January 23, 2021, I went to the washroom to throw up. I went on to throw up four times, pure black vile. When I was finished getting sick. I wiped my mouth and told myself to call 911. I also reminded myself that if the emerge doctors want to send you home. You must put your foot down and just say NO! I did, and that's how I began to have happy days with a hernia.

CHAPTER 18
Happy Days with Hitial Hernia

The date was January 24, 2021. The time was 10 p.m., and yet again, I was in the back of an ambulance. As one of the EMTs tried to get my information, I told him I was exhausted from going to the hospital and getting a band-aid to fix the problem. I went on to say to him that no matter what they say tonight in emerge, "I was going to have to put my foot down and demand to be fixed; if they refuse, then I just might die at home in the next little while." After the EMTs gave them the report and my pulse and blood pressure stats, I lay there in sickbay waiting to see what the doctor was going to say... After having X-rays ordered, the on-call emerge doctor told me that I have a pretty large hiatal hernia, which explains why I cannot keep food down... The Doc says, "here at the hospital, we don't have the division to help you. You have to go to another hospital." I nodded to say Okay, here we go again, they're going to send me home, and my family will hear about my death one night while eating dinner and watching the news, I thought. As I spoke up to the doctor, I reminded him to look at my chart, and there was one thing I wanted him to look at on my chart. I wanted him to see firsthand with hi6666s own eyes just how many times I have been to the hospital

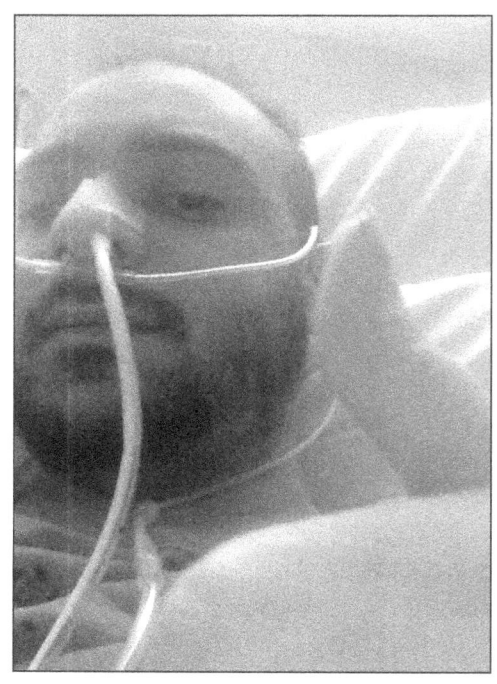

24 hours before hernia surgery, January 2021.

in the past year for the same reason of throwing up blood. I kindly said to the on-call doctor, "Listen, doc, I have suffered enough through this; if I am kept in the hospital for a few days and sent home, you will find me here again next month for the same issues. Help me, get this hernia out of me, please; I can't even keep food down; I don't need you to put a band-aid on the problem; I need this fixed."

He then said, "Okay. Let me see what the other hospital says about what to do..." After waiting for 30 minutes, the doctor returned to me and told me that I would be transported to Victoria Hospital tomorrow afternoon in the thoracic department for emergency surgery. The E.R. doctor also said they would keep me in the hospital overnight with IV fluids and anti-nausea medication to avoid getting sick again. When I finished with the doctor, I called my brother Angelo to tell him what was happening and that I was heading in for surgery in only a few hours. "Finally, all of these problems will eventually be over soon. Angelo, then reminded me to get some sleep and that I am to call him tomorrow before the surgery..." I asked him to call me in a few hours post-surgery if I wake up because I will probably be out of it and unable to contact you. Call the recovery room, and they will let you know everything I said...

At 1:30 p.m., the nurses of University Hospital came to me and said, "to prep you for surgery; we have to insert a G-Tube up your nose." At this point, I was so tired; I did not care, so I just said, whatever you got to do, just do it, anything that helps me get this fixed, I will do."

The nurses left to get the supplies for the G-tube. When the nurse came back, he gave me very special instructions. "Anthony, here is a cup of water with a straw; do it right away when I tell you to drink with the straw. As you're drinking the water, I will feed the tube into your nose, down into your stomach." I am sorry if my body tries to reject you because I have CP, and I often don't have things shoved in my nose. He responded by saying, Ha, no one does; it can be very uncomfortable...."

As the G-Tube was getting inserted into my nose, the first thing that came to mind was, "there has to be a simpler way than the caveman way. Getting a G-Tube just put in your nose so it can go down into your stomach almost seems too easy, and it doesn't involve any form of technology at all and the last time I checked the calendar, the year wasn't 1921, but it was the year 2021. The nurse was indeed right; getting the tube inserted into your nose wasn't very relaxing at all... At first, when they began with the insertion, I wanted to mule kick them, but then I realized that if I kicked them in the nose and they started to bleed, then both our noses would be hurting, and that didn't help anybody...

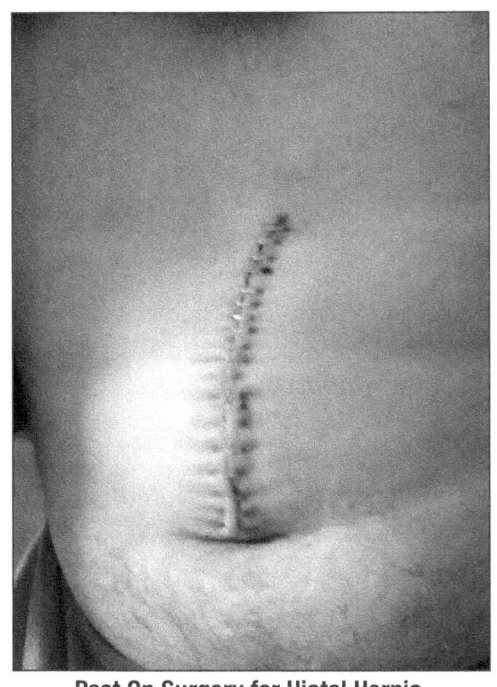

Post Op Surgery for Hiatal Hernia. January 31, 2021.

After the nurse was done with the G-Tube, they realized they had put it in the wrong location, and therefore, they had removed it and tried to insert it again. I was none too pleased, but like I said in the beginning, *"I am willing to do whatever it takes to get me on the operating table." At 2 p.m. January 25, 2021,* I was transferred from University Hospital to Victoria Hospital's fifth floor C wing. At 3 p.m., I was signing papers to have emergency surgery, and at 5 p.m. that same day, I was wheeled into the operating room. Moments before I entered the operating room, I spoke with the anesthesiologist or, as I would like to call him, the medicine man. He told me what kind of drugs they would use to put me under, and then he asked me if I had any questions. I only had one, "Do you need my weight?" He responded by saying, "No, we have it on file. Okay," let's do the surgery, I thought.

Before, I would take a medically induced nap; the surgeons had me sit up so they could give me a needle in my spine. They informed me how to bend my neck, sit forward and look at the wall. I did this so that they could inject the epidural into my spine for freezing and future pain management. After the surgery, I was rolled into the recovery area, where I would lay out cold for three and half hours. The surgery happened at 5:30 p.m. and wrapped up at about 9:30 p.m. When I awoke from my slumber, I glanced at the clock, and the time was 1:15 a.m., January 26, 2021. When I had a sense of where I was, I had two nurses beside me, coaching me to breathe. They struggled for a good 25 minutes to get me to breathe; all I wanted to do was go to sleep; I kept fading in and out. Finally, the nurse by my left shoulder screamed out, "I think we gave him too much anesthesia; we need to turn it down." As I looked ahead, there was the nursing desk, and apparently, my brother Angelo called to see if I was still alive and if I made it through surgery OK. The nurse spoke to my brother, saying to him that the surgery went well; he's just starting to wake up now and then he will be transported to a room upstairs,

As I was transported to my room, the time on the wall said 2 a.m. The night from 2 a.m. onward to 8 p.m. was a blur the first night; the medication was a big reason; God Bless that old pain pump of mine. The first official day post-surgery was extremely tiring, and it seemed that all I wanted to do was nap. Now there is something I want my readers to know just because I felt sleepy for the first 48 hours. It doesn't mean I had terrible nurses. The nurses were extremely pleasant the nurses were great people and even carried on a short conversation with me when I was awake from me in and out dozing off episodes. They all did their job extremely well and managed to even keep me comfortable. On day two, I had a little more awareness of where I was. The medical team came into my room to see me on day two. Each team member was great.

Some of the nurses tipped off the doctors and let them know that I was about to work for the London Knights Hockey Team before the pandemic happened... I am sure that is why I often felt spoiled because they wanted me to work for the Knights once again. Also, on the second day, the surgeon came in to speak with me about the operation. He said the surgery was a success. Your hernia was huge, and I had to repair your throat as well. Now being the type of person I am, I am not one to shy away from asking the tough questions. I asked the doctor, "Could the hernia have killed me if it ruptured differently." Yes, he said, you would have never even made it to the hospital had it explode in your stomach." Wow, I said, you saved my life, thanks, Doctor RN."

The next day the team of doctors again came Into my room to see how I was doing. I said I felt like a big grizzly bear pawed my abs. The wound was closed with 17 staples. The Doctors would visit me every day for 18 days while I was there at Victoria Hospital in acute care. For the first five days, I couldn't eat a thing. I was on a fast. I once asked the doctors when I could eat, and they told me they would give me food when I was able to fart. I didn't fart for seven days. My stomach was trying its best to recover from the recent trauma. On the fourth day of seeing the doctors, the Nurse Practitioner asks the famous question," Anthony, did you fart yet?" I replied by saying NO! Give me some beans, Andrew, and then I will fart." He laughed as he went on to see the next patient. After not passing wind, the doctors ordered a protein and electrolyte pump on day five. I was scheduled to be on the pump for just 48 hours. After two days, at 11 p.m., I passed some gas, and the doctors were so happy about that news because it meant that they could take the G-Tube out of my nose. After being on the Total Parenteral Nutrition bag or, in simpler terms, TPN bag, which helps supports a patient's protein-electrolyte balance, I was on the TPN bag for two days; I went to the bathroom about 11 times in one day. One of the nurses watching over me that day was concerned about what she saw in my bowel movement. She decided to send a sample to the lab, and a few hours later that day, I was informed by Andrew that I was infected with *Clostridioides difficile* or C-diff.

What C-Diff is for people that don't know it is a bacterial infection in the bowels that, if not treated properly, can cause a severe case of dehydration because you have a severe case of diarrhea. Thankfully I wasn't in the care of just any group of nurses. I had only the best group of nurses looking after me. They did a great job not making my C-Diff diagnosis a life-threatening big deal.

I joked with the nurses about my infection, saying, "I guess the one good thing about pooping your pants in the hospital is you get your own room." I followed that up with the line, "you guys and gals don't have to get all dressed up for me with special gowns and gloves, but I appreciate it." However, if it's all the same for all of you nurses, can someone please tell me when the pooping will stop. It's embarrassing." The nurses reminded me that it's not your fault. The bacteria in your bowels are causing you to go so frequently." The doctors ordered that the best way to treat the infection in my bowels was to put me on a liquid drug called vancomycin. After 12 days, the infection was gone, but the idea of where to send me was still up in the air. So, during the pooping problem, I levelled with Andrew and asked him to get me a transfer to Parkwood Hospital for some rehab because I hadn't had the strength to walk in three years... The doctors agreed that sending me to a rehab facility was perhaps the best thing for me, considering the medical struggles. That being said, I did have just excellent therapists at Vic Hospital "Carolynn and Jo. You're the best, and you both deserve gold star awards for the year." To Carolyn and Jo's credit they took someone like me and that had me up and walking. I was walking slow yes, but the important thing to remember here is that I was walking and personally for myself, I felt that was a huge accomplishment. Thanks Carolyn and Jo for everything. On February 12, 2021, I was transferred to Parkwood Hospital at 8 a.m. It was a decision I would later regret for the rest of my life.

CHAPTER 19
Parkwood Prison

Originally the first couple drafts of this book had this chapter under a different title. In the beginning, I thought to name this chapter Perseverance Begins at Parkwood, but after my experience with the hospital, I felt a more appropriate title for this chapter was Parkwood Prison. I will give my readers a warning; at times, writing this chapter may seem like I am Frank Costanza airing his grievances at the Festivus table, but I promise to all who read this chapter and to all who are reading this book: Everything you are about to read in this chapter is entirely factual; I have legal documents and audio recordings to back up my claims.

As I said earlier, I was transferred to Parkwood Hospital for what I thought would be eight weeks of rehab to be prepared for surgery on my hip that was separated. Initially, I was under the impression that the idea of going to Parkwood Hospital was for rehab, I thought that's what Victoria Hospital and the therapists Carolynn and Jo were getting ready for, so I would be an acceptable candidate for their rehab. To show transparency, that's precisely why I was receiving any therapy at Vic Hospital because, as a patient, I had to meet a certain level of standards to be considered for their MSK rehab program. On February 12, 2021, my stay at Parkwood began...

The first day was typical; I met a group of doctors, a dietitian and a team of therapists. Meeting the dietitian was necessary for the surgery I just had on my stomach. Post-surgery I was put on a special diet for 60 days. The type of diet that I was put on was an esophageal-soft diet. In layman's terms, it just means my food had to be puréed. When I met Dr. Natalie Needles the following Friday, I was given a discharge date of March 16. When given the date, I strongly contested their decision. I told them in no uncertain terms that I would NOT be ready to return home.

"I haven't walked in three years, and no matter the therapy, I will need more time than a month." They went on to say, "well,

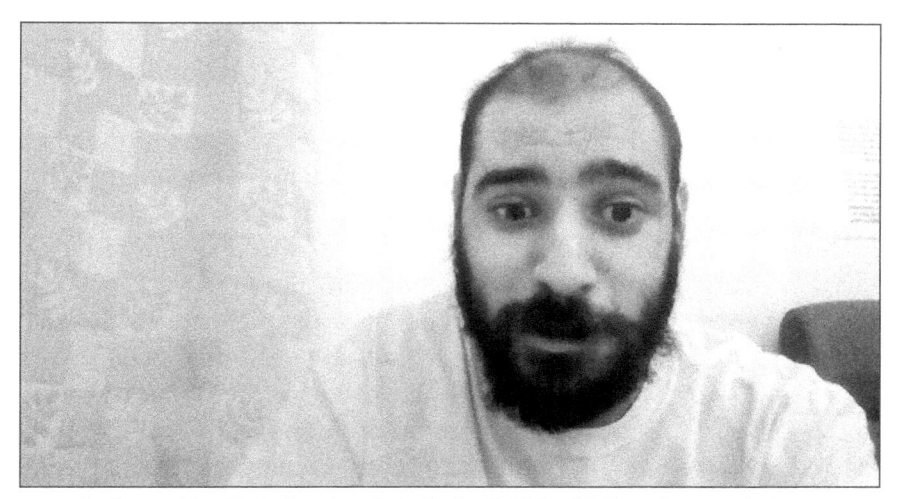

Parkwood Institute London Ontario April 2021. 60 Days in my rehab stay wondering when they're going to release me.

typically, we only keep patients here for three weeks. That's the rules." I said, "I don't care about the rules; the rules just changed because I have different care needs than your average patient. I went on to tell them that I didn't plan on having ulcers, hernias and dislocated hips for the past three years, but they all happened, and I had to accommodate my life to get the best care possible through a difficult time." You're wrong to make a snap decision to make me leave in one month just so it's convenient for you so that it can free up a bed. None of these medical issues is convenient for me, but I solider through it because I am determined to see things through."

The reason I highly contested my discharge was for various reasons; first of all, I was put on a special diet by my surgical team, and the last time I walked down the aisle of my local FRESHCO, they didn't have a special food aisle in their store that said esophageal soft diet food located in aisle seven. Secondly, I knew that even though I was not a medical doctor, I didn't need special eyeglasses to see that I needed much help rebuilding my lost muscle. When I brought that to their attention, they told me they don't have that kind of time. When I was told this by their resident therapist Sarah Scappers. I replied, "Take a minute to listen to yourself, this hospital is a rehab hospital, and you're telling a patient that we don't have the time to rehab you for three months. She said that's right only because you are in too much pain." I nodded and agreed and said yes, I am in pain but look at the bigger picture here. Pain is a part of the process. I have to be in shape and healthy enough for upcoming surgery." I would rather be in pain and somewhat mobile than the complete opposite: sitting in my wheelchair doing nothing and loading up on pills every four hours."

Dealing with that team, I faced the same struggles and red tape barriers every day. My efforts in physical therapy were beyond anyone's expectations. When asked to walk the parallel bars, I walked them backwards and frontwards several times in different sessions. When asked to work on the hand bicycle for a few sessions, I did 15 minutes each time. I did 15 minutes for different sessions when asked to use the stepper machine. I became so frustrated with the physical therapy department video evidence for social media, just in case people wondered why I wast's a treatment that I decided to provide still not walking constantly?

I decided to take measures into my hands because I wanted to prove a point to the surgeons and the general public. The reason I felt I had a lacklustre rehabilitation is that for the most of my therapy sessions at Parkwood, when I wasn't on the machines, I was getting stretched out by most of the therapists that were supposed to be hands-on and from my experience with them, it didn't take me long to discover that not a single person could care less.

I became so frustrated with the physical therapy team at Parkwood Hospital that I decided to provide Facebook with video evidence of my efforts in my therapy sessions. I chose to provide video evidence of my rehab sessions for two reasons. I wanted to show others that the reason I was not walking wasn't for lack of effort. The only reason I wasn't walking as best as I could during my rehab sessions was that the physical therapists inside the walls of Parkwood Hospital's fifth-floor MSK Program are entirely incompetent.

A number of them were either on their phones sending text messages or on the computer sending emails. My Parkwood roommate caught the one therapist looking at porn on the computer while he was supposed to be counting and stretching the patient out. After I heard and saw that myself, I thought to myself, "well, that about sums up their attitude towards the rehab of patients."

Nice job, Tyler! Way to take advantage of the system. I even told Tyler to "stop going on the computer while you're working with me just to look at women's breasts. If you want to do that, fine, do it on your own damn time and stop wasting mine while I'm trying to get better."

Finally, about a month into my recovery, the medical team realized that I wouldn't go anywhere, and I was prepared to take them to court if I had to. They eventually concluded that they couldn't send me home because my home was a disaster with vomit everywhere from the ulcers and stomach hernia. Also, the team believed I would require too much help from local community support if I went home, and rightly so. I backed them into a corner, and they had to figure out what to do. I had a phone consult with my orthopedic surgeon. I told Dr. Ortho that the hospital wanted to send me home, but I didn't feel like I could go home in a safe manner, given that my hip was separated. I asked the surgeon, "would there be any way that my surgery can be moved up, so they don't discharge me foolishly." Doctor Ortho said, "let me check in with your other surgeon Dr. Esphofo to see if you are medically cleared to have another surgery." The Parkwood medical team got back to me and told me that I would be having surgery on March 25, 2021...

I was beyond thrilled with the news... I was informed of this on March 17. As happy as I was to hear the news that the surgery would take place, Parkwood Hospital had a way of throwing me a curveball and ruining any joy that I had leading up to surgery... The date was March 24, 2021. I was called into a room filled with social workers, and they wanted to figure out where to place me post-surgery because they felt that there was no way I could be rehabbed. "Time out..." I want to make readers aware that I will do my best to explain what went on in the closed-door meeting to show complete transparency. I met with many social workers in this meeting, and I guess I was supposed to have a conference call with the doctor and my parents. They made excuses about calling the doctor another time right off the bat. However, the social workers felt led to call my parents still and inform them that they thought it best that I go into a long-term care setting. I said, "if the doctor won't be called, then there is no reason to involve my parents, to employ your sick tactics so that I go against my mother and father on the phone. I told them both my parents are very sick and don't speak for me; I am a big boy, I will speak for myself..."

At this point, I was getting irritated with them, and I said, "I am not going to fall for your bullshit games. Try to play me against my mother so you can have veto power is disgusting, and all of you should be ashamed of yourselves." They said, "Dr. Malice has a good plan, and we think it's the best option." I responded to them, saying, "I don't give a shit what doctor Dr. Malice has to say. He is not the one cutting me open, and he is not the one I have a signed medical contract. Dr. Ortho and I agree that he deals with this kind of stuff every day, and I will follow his instructions, not the thoughts of Dr. Malice. If you all disagree with what my orthopedic surgeon wants to do, I will be more than happy to walk out of the room right now, and you all can go to hell" I then left the room. Even though I was furious when I left the room, I was pretty happy the surgery was the next day, so I didn't have to put up with their nonsense anymore. To put it in context, just so all my readers understand, I knew I was getting cut open in 24 hours, and I was excited about that because it meant that I could escape the chaos of Parkwood Prison. I was so happy; it felt like I was going on vacation.

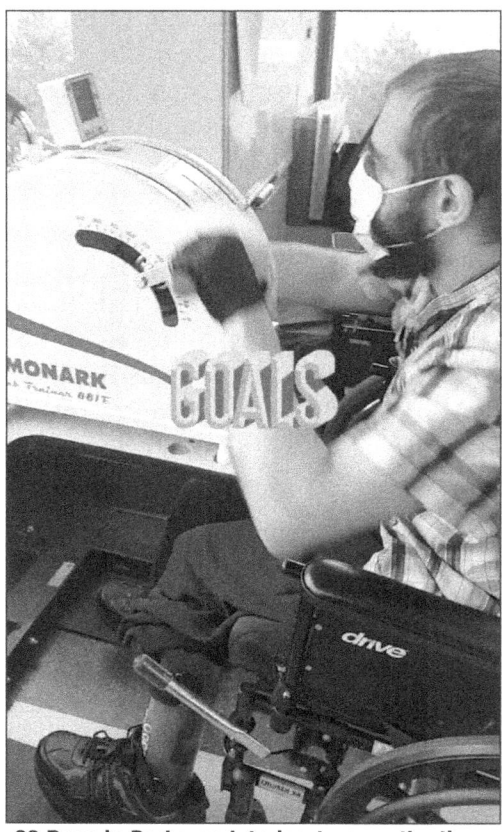

90 Days in Parkwood, trying to pass the time.

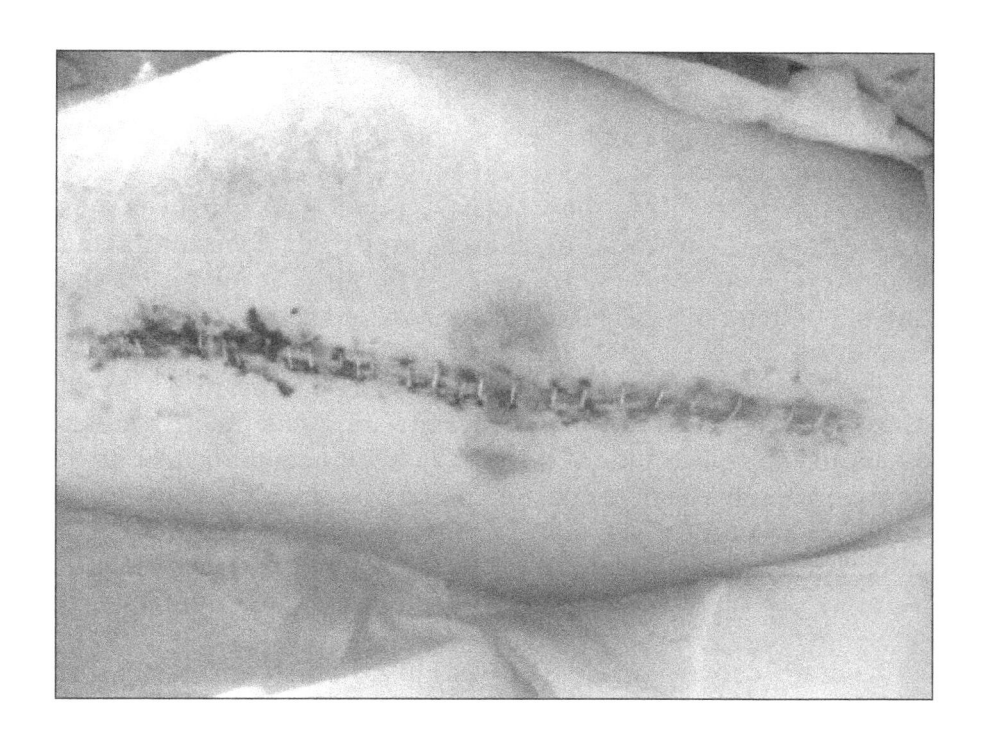

CHAPTER 20
A New Hip at 36

On March 25, 2021, a day that I would remember as the day that I got carved up more than a Thanksgiving turkey in November. Nothing that happened on that day was ordinary. I arrived at University Hospital at 8:30 a.m. When I arrived in the pre surgery area I was asked the typical medical rhetoric that a patient usually is asked before going into the operating room. After the hospital understood who my emergency contacts were and what blood type I was, the surgeon came to visit me for a short time, during his short visit Dr. Ortho asked me if I was ready to have the surgery? I simply, smiled and laughed and said, "Let's make history." He then nodded with approval and then I was wheeled into a room full of nurses to receive another needle in the spine. The nurses were extremely nice to me. Some of them, asked them what I hoped for after this surgery? At that time, I had nothing to lose. The only thing I could tell them was the absolute truth.

"I'm approaching 36 years old and my parents are in their early '70s for me getting another scar is nothing new to me, but I want the surgery to provide a good outcome. When I am able to get on my feet again, I want to show my parents that their sacrifices weren't wasted. I don't want them to go to their deathbeds thinking that they failed because they couldn't fix this disability." When my minor deformity gets fixed many surgeons can help future generations of the same problem."

The nurses that were around me that day and heard me speak those words looked at each other and said, "this young kid has goals and a good attitude to boot." As I left the room to be brought in the operating room, the doctors if I had anything to say. I simply said, "Please let me say thank you to the surgeon for doing this surgery for me." Dr. Ortho heard me thank him for his time in preforming the surgery. He being most modest simply replied, "No problem, Tony."

After the surgery was over, I would be the first to admit that it felt nice not having to scream in pain, just the thought that they had the idea to freeze my left surgical leg was a blessing and I am sure it made it much easier on my nighttime nurses and any in the future for at least the first 48 hours. After the second day past, I asked for pills. Now my readers must understand that asking for pain medication is certainly difficult to ask, because I lead a straight edge life, which means, I don't take drugs, drink or smoke. However, I have my own rules, I'm not an idiot or a prude. If my body of mine is healing from surgery then I understand that there is a certain realization that you must stay on top of your pain management at least for the first few days post-surgery. On day three of being at UH the surgeon came into see me and he said the surgery couldn't have gone as well as it did. He was extremely pleased with the outcome.

He then spoke to me and said, I would be returning to Parkwood Hospital for rehab, I kindly protested mentioning to Dr. Ortho that rehab will not go well there when I return. I told the doctor that Parkwood Hospital isn't interested in rehabbing me at all. I followed that by saying, Parkwood Hospital's focus is get me to return under their care just so they can place me in long term care.

I went on, to express my complete distain for being placed in long term care if it's not under my conditions. To be clear, I wasn't against going into long term care if it had what I required. However, if a facility didn't have what I needed than I would fight the hospital tooth and nail with lawyers advocating for disability rights. The doctors wanted to remind me, that they will make sure that I get the rehab necessary to go back home. As much as I hoped things would be different when I returned to Parkwood Hospital, nothing changed, and I began to see the complete incompetence of the physical therapy and occupational therapy departments. When I returned to the hospital, I call Parkwood Prison and after much discussion about the new type of rehab I would need, it didn't take long for me to see that the ladies that were "working on my rehab program didn't have the knowledge to look after kids on a school playground.

Therefore it is in my highly expressed opinion that the physical therapists working with me on the fifth floor do not have the proper knowledge or expertise to begin my rebuilding process. In fact, the more I participated in any form of therapy with this group, the more I began to see the exercise aficionados began to treat patients in their care like cars going through a McDonald's drive thru. In fact, there's really only one major difference between a McDonald's drive thru worker and the physical therapists at Parkwood Hospital. The guys and gals that are stationed at your local McDonald's drive thru window actually have manners. Not one of the therapists within the walls of Parkwood Hospital weren't even fit enough to tie my shoelaces, so if that was the case and given my previous experiences with them just weeks prior to the surgery does anybody really have to question why I just couldn't trust not only the therapists and doctors, but even the nurses walked around acting above the law.

CHAPTER 21
Doctors of Doubt Disabling Your Rights

As I returned to the horrible hospital, it didn't take me long to discover that the monkeys in the therapy department wasn't going to rehab me. Whenever I was told to stop doing therapy after 10 minutes on the hand bike or NU step, I told the therapists. I will not listen to any of you because just working out 10 minutes a day wasn't helping anybody. It was just moving the ensembled line along to the next patient, and I was not okay with that at all... I knew that if I was going to get better, I had to find a good balance between what I could do and if I was sometimes hurting, I would see myself not saying a word because I hated taking any medication. I didn't allow myself to take the prescribed medication often because, after a while, the nurses at Parkwood Hospital seemed to be pushing the meds on me to keep me in a subedited state of unawareness. The truth behind the pill-popping propaganda is that every day I was scheduled to take Tylenol four times a day at a dosage of 650 each time.

In addition to being on four dosses of acetaminophen per day, I was also on muscle relaxers and hydro-morph for serve pain. I was on 30 milligrams a day of the muscle relaxer known as Baclofen. I couldn't even tell you why I was on that drug. However, if you talk to the doctors at Parkwood Hospital, they will tell you that the reason I am on such medications like the muscle relaxers has a lot to do with cerebral palsy spasms, but myself and you, the reader, know the truth. It's all about supporting big pharma. I am against being on muscle relaxers because even though it's true that sometimes I do have spasms, the spasms don't need to be treated with medication because they are not debilitating or stopping me from living my life. Aside from being a patient at Parkwood Hospital, I have never been on muscle relaxers ever in my life. The idea to have me try muscle relaxers came from the brain of Dr. Natalie Needles because she is supposed to be a specialist in the treatment of generalized cerebral palsy.

With regards to Dr. Natalie Needles, she may have a very young-looking face and a ponytail, but, in my opinion, it doesn't excuse her from making decisions without consulting me first.

After a few months of going through the motions of rehab, Dr. Needles and her pretentious ponytail pulled me into a room that just informed me out of the blue that they would be stopping my rehab. Getting that kind of news was extremely upsetting because as much as I was trying to put in the effort to be as healthy as I could be from a walking perspective. The truth is simply related to the horrible hospital known as Parkwood. I had very realistic goals, goals that took time to manifest, and the truth is, the hospital and their rehab program took my goals into account and flat out told me that's not what we are here for. Even though I made my goals very clear, it is evident that they were not going to help me. On several occasions, I questioned their medical expertise on how a man like myself should walk steadily with a walker after just two weeks of therapy? Their very far-sided reasoning was about getting the next patient in the hospital. When Dr. Thorton Malice came back on service in the summertime, his idea was to set me up with a new pair of leg braces and then hand me off to the social workers so they could plant me in a long-term care facility. After receiving my leg braces on May 6, 2021, I was then scheduled to meet with the social workers about where I should go upon my discharge.

On Friday, May 7, 2021, a day, a piece of me died, and in reality, it's something I haven't even recovered from simply because I was in a constant war with the hospital about my rights. On Friday, May 7, 2021, it was announced that my friend, pastor and mentor had died. Immediately because I saw the posting on social media, I thought this was a joke because the pastor was old. Reverend Ernest Angley was 99 years old, and he was such a mentor to me that even though I was in the hospital, he stayed in contact with me throughout the whole time by way of an email. When I developed ulcers and later hernia, he was there. If I had an urgent question about classes and the bible, he always took time to see me when I was taking Bible College classes in Ohio. As he was affectionally referred to as those who knew him, Reverend taught me so much.

Starting point: It was because of the Reverend Ernest Angley and constantly communicating with him through a terrible time, I decided that when it came time to design some braces, they were going to be designed with the Reverend in mind. I decided to design my leg braces with the face of Reverend Angley on my braces, but not only his face; I decided to make the design a bit more personal. I took one of my favourite books by Reverend Angley. I allowed the orthopedic specialists to bring the book cover of his autobiography, *Hurry Friday*, and wear that on my braces. From a personal standpoint, as it relates to myself, there was no way of knowing that I would get the mounts on the sixth of May and then hear about the Reverend's passing the very next day.

There was no way of knowing that I would get the tragic news of the passing of Rev on the same day that I would get my leg braces. It was bittersweet.

His passing affected everybody that knew him, and it was unexpected; I mean, as members of the church, we learned how old he was, but he sure didn't act his age, and everyone was more than excited that he was going to be turning 100 years old just two months later. After receiving the extremely sentimental leg braces, Dr. Malice passed me off to the sharks or social workers as their job title reflects their ambitions.

The hospital and the social workers wanted to dictate their narrative right away, saying that I needed to go to a long-term care facility. I agreed with the conditions be-

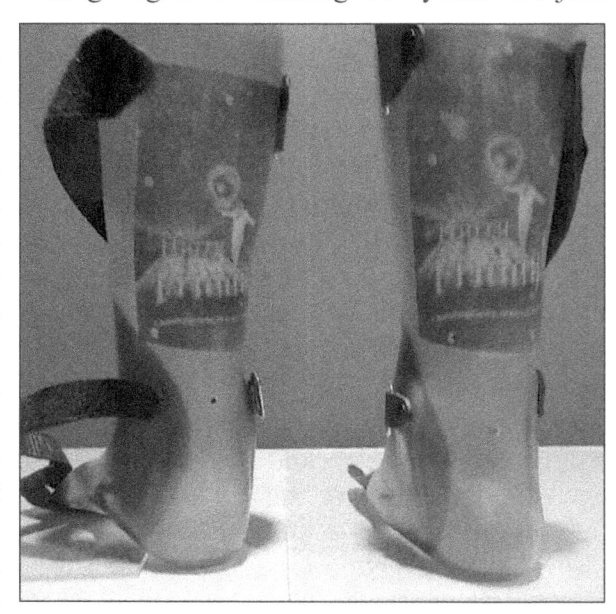

Hurry Friday Leg Braces. A tribute to the life and legacy of Reverend Ernest Angley.

cause I knew I was in no shape to return home, for me to be willing to agree to long-term home for a short while until I had news on when my hip surgery will be scheduled for a full hip replacement. After all, that was the reason I was given my first hip surgery. Dr. Ortho removed the steel plates so I could have a new hip in the future because I had what doctors called osteoarthritis, and it's in my genes, and the only way to fix that is a full hip replacement.

After getting my braces and finishing my rehab, I was still in a lot of pain, and the resident doctor who came on in relief of Dr. Needles and Dr. Malice was Doctor Rachel Rhetoric. Before I go any further, I should clarify that doctors' names mentioned in this book are not their actual real names. I named each doctor based on their behaviour and how stupid each white coat person truly was. Dr. Malice was named because of his constant need to feel far superior to his patients. I named him Dr. Malice because his behaviour led me to believe he practiced medicine with arrogance and malicious intent. The name Doctor Natalie Needles came about because she was familiar with Botox treatment injections for the treatment of cerebral palsy. Yes, as a man, I have had my fair share of Botox injections because initially, I was made to believe that these injections were supposed to help me somehow.

Both Dr. Needles and Dr. Rhetoric were quick to jab me with needles because they felt that having these injections was much better than having a full hip replacement. When I look back on their medical observations suggesting I should get Botox vs an actual hip replacement is rather idiotic at best, and that's me being kind to them. When someone with my cerebral palsy condition comes along and requires a total hip replacement to live a life without pain, another group of doctors say that I should forget about getting hip surgery. Still, I should focus my energy on getting injection after injection. I am not one to say no to a trial of medicine if it has a good result in the end. When Doctors explain some experimental medical practices and trials, I would be one of the first persons to say yes to a specialized treatment if I felt that an experiment or trials proves to be in my best interest than I am fully on board for anything after a short discussion with the doctor performing the treatment.

I named the other doctor in this story Rachel Rhetoric because she was a doctor that went by the book in every way; she even had the librarian glasses firmly placed on her nose to prove it. Every time she and I talked about my care, she would stick to the same medical jargon about "the hospital policy." I was the patient to say, fuck the hospital's policy and look out for the patient's care first. When I couldn't agree with doctors about rehab and advocating for myself when it came to getting the best care possible, the doctors would send me back to the social workers to wear down my stance.

Given the past opposition, I had with these doctors prior to my return to Parkwood Institute, I felt if the doctor was just going to give me a mundane response, then I would be the type of patient that would openly contest them by saying fuck the hospital policy give me real answers.

I also want to be clear that my demands to be entered into a long-term home were very simple. I wanted them to cover the cost because I didn't ever want to give up my home so that I could pay two and a half grand per month while I waited to go home. I also wanted to be sure that there would be a meal plan within this facility. I also wanted to be sure that wherever I ended up, this place had a place I could work out because if the rehab hospital refused to keep me healthy for the subsequent surgery, I would take it upon myself to do it. I mean, by no means am I Billy Blanks or Chuck Norris, but I would give one hell of a shot to rebuild my body from the ground up, even if it meant that I had to do this on my own. One thing I did before I left Parkwood Hospital was I went to see my orthopedic surgeon about what I could do in the future because I had informed him that I had a trial-and-error performance at Parkwood Hospital, and that's putting it in a nice way without just flat out saying that my time within the rehab hospital was complete bullshit and truly felt like a waste of time.

However, before I left Parkwood Hospital, I got it across to Dr. Ortho that although I very much appreciated what he was able to do for me, I insisted on perhaps when we look at getting the final hip surgery done than perhaps, we should come together with a plan to send me to a decent rehab centre. I made it clear to doctor Ortho that I didn't ever want to return to Parkwood Hospital; I wanted to go to a facility where I would get the most out of the facility in general. I made a commitment to my surgeon, saying that if he did the best he could when replacing my hip, I would give my all as long as I went to the best rehab facility to support what I needed to help me prepare for life post-new hip. In the past, Parkwood has said on multiple occasions that I shouldn't get hope of wanting to walk again. I pleaded with my surgeon to put a referral to the Toronto Rehab Centre.

CHAPTER 22
Tenacity in Toronto

When I informed Doctor Ortho about my sincere intentions to pursue going to Toronto Rehab Centre, I did so with the utmost research. From my perspective, here's how it looks on paper. Parkwood had a chance to make a difference; I gave the staff ample time to get me well enough. However, I believe that the medical team within the walls of their hospital believes I set unrealistic expectations. As far as myself goes being the patient going through this ordeal, I decided to pick the Toronto Rehab Centre because I wanted fresh eyes on my recovery. How could something like that benefit me? Well, I will only say this in passing. The city of London had many years of getting me well, however, there comes a time in a man's life where decisions have to be made and I personally thought that I had outgrown the city of London in terms the treatment of my Cerebral Palsy for the remainder of my adult life. I felt having a fresh pair of eyes on my condition wouldn't at all hurt. I had to look at it as a simple transition from childhood to manhood. The same tactics used as a child to treat my condition I felt would not work because the progression of the illness changes with age and time, ie: a build-up of arthritis in the hips over time. I believe the apostle Paul said it best in the New Testament as he addressed a letter written to the Corinthians.

"When I was a child, I spake as a child, I understood as a child, I thought as a child: but when I became a man, I put away childish things." 1 Corinthians 13:11, King James Version.

The need for personal growth is again brought to the forefront in the book of Hebrews. Hebrews 5:12-14, King James Version.

> [12] For when for the time ye ought to be teachers, ye have need that one teach you again which be the first principles of the oracles of God; and are become such as have need of milk, and not of strong meat.
>
> [13] For every one that useth milk is unskilful in the word of

righteousness: for he is a babe.

[14] But strong meat belongeth to them that are of full age, even those who by reason of use have their senses exercised to discern both good and evil.

Maybe if the doctors at Parkwood Hospital spent a little less time being brainwashed in pessimism and a little more time studying how to be optimistic, more patients would leave that hospital with a feeling of time well spent because they worked hard to achieve a goal. As a medical patient dealing with my physical condition, I have no problem seeking new tactics if there are benefits. If I were to go back to Parkwood Hospital, it would be better to have my legs cut off than give the morons charge over my physical health again.

CHAPTER 23
These Bones Can Live!

At the Toronto Rehab Centre I am very keen on being open and transparent with the medical team about my goals because ultimately that's truly what it is really all about. The focus is long standing personal independence for a better quality of life. The question becomes how can the surgery and rehab help me establish physical independence even if I have to use walking aids to manage it. I believe Parkwood believes that I am out to prove a point. That's not entirely true. Despite public opinion and perception, I don't plan to go to rehab with the mindset of being just like a Rocky Balboa-type character. I have a small secret the world must be made of right here and now. I will go on record to say that even though sometimes I act determined and courageous, I am not Superman. Having that mindset is the elephant in the room or an outrageous and unrealistic goal that could never truly and physically be achieved. I believe the world needs to focus more time on being original. I don't want to be the next Rocky; I am okay with being Anthony Franco Sicilia. Besides, I am a lot tougher. Don't believe me? Every scar on my body would cause you to believe me in my love and hate relationship with CP. My parents were utterly relentless in fixing or repairing me because they wanted me to be accepted in society; they also wanted to have the same opportunities, even though I love them for their effort. As a man full of age, I've understood the simple reality that people can fight and beat cancer. However with me, I have very different challenges. I have realized that I don't need to conquer cerebral palsy because, in this world, it's better to stand up and stand out. That's how someone with my disability makes a difference, inspires the public, and challenges the overall perception of dealing with people's physical challenges. If someone like myself can understand that it's okay to evolve and grow physically by keeping up with therapy constantly, then that's how disfigured bones can live. These can be achieved by adapting to physical differences post-surgery.

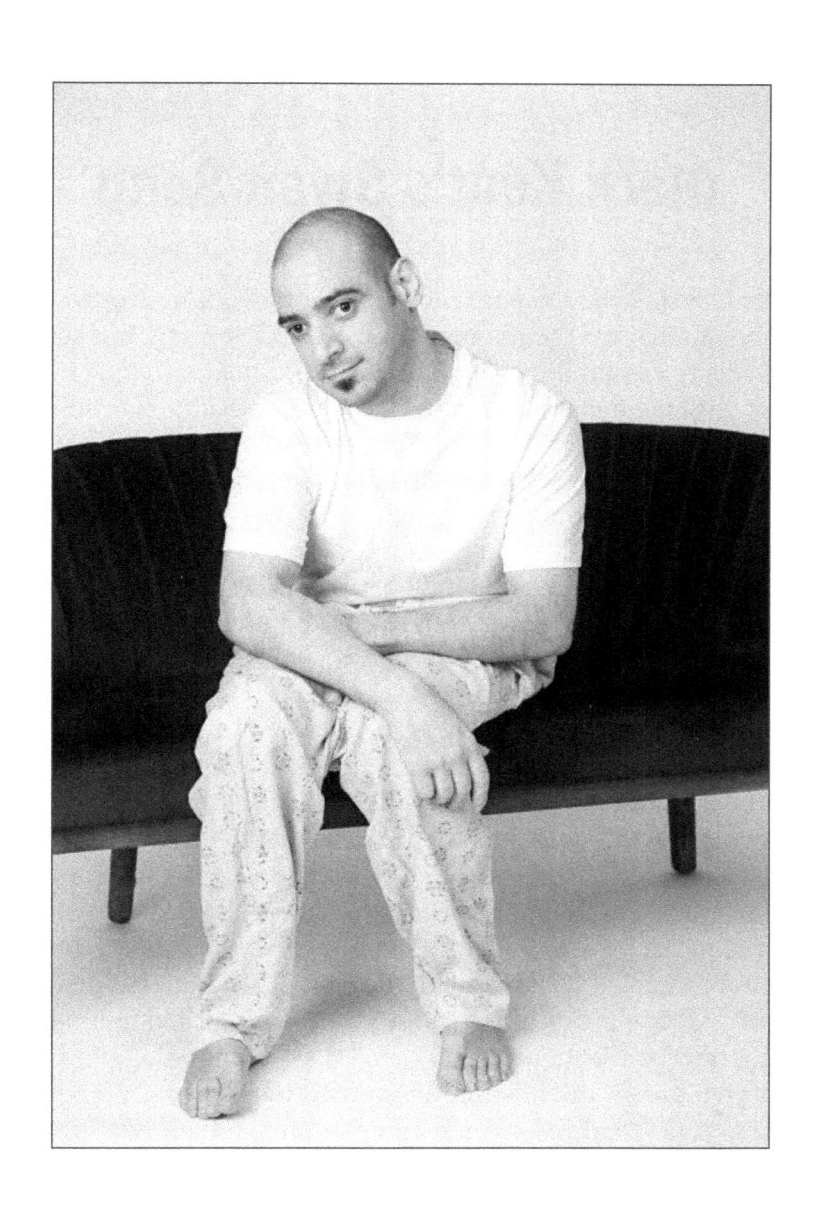

CHAPTER 24
Clark Kent's Swan Song

The idea for this chapter came about on April 8, 2022, around 3 p.m. I had just gotten off the phone with Doctor Ortho, my hip surgeon, at University Hospital in London, Ontario, Canada. He had a phone consult with me that afternoon to let me know that he was still planning on doing surgery for me in the coming months. He was waiting for an opening in his schedule. "I said, Okay, that's fine. I am in no rush." Did I lie to the great Doctor Ortho? I prefer to say that I stretched the truth a little. In reality, I was eager to have hip replacement surgery, but I did not want to make the doctor feel uncomfortable or act in a way that seemed hasty or indecisive. I have the utmost respect for any of the surgeons I have worked with on my skeletal system. While I had him on the phone, I asked him a question while still in the hot seat.

Where would you like me to do rehab post-surgery doc?

He said I think it's best to go to Parkwood for a short stint in the recovery and rehab program. I quickly thought to myself, NO! Please don't send me to the Ellis Island of Healthcare. After we exchanged our goodbyes to each other, I quickly wondered why in the world he would send me back to Parkwood Prison, given my recent and utter disdain for them? I had to quickly figure out a way to get out of this position. After all, I didn't want to go to Ellis Island again on the 5th floor and be a patient inside their MSK program again, only to get thrown out of the hospital in zip ties by two or three security guards that failed at Strongman competitions in their not-so-distant past. I knew from a personal standpoint that if I became a patient on the fifth floor, once again, things wouldn't go well. I knew if I saw Doctor Malice's face again, his arrogance would put me in a challenging position. Scenario #1: I walk up to the doctor and attack him like a scene from S.E. Hinton's *The Outsiders*.

I didn't want to jeopardize my health by not staying focused on the real reason I was sent there. So, with that in mind, I called up the head of my family, Papa Tony, and I knew he would understand how to deal with the situation that I presented because for my family and me, it wasn't the first moron that my family and I dealt with that had no hope of me walking again. I knew I needed to remain calm and research to see if I could find a loophole. As I was on the phone with Papa Tony, he told me, "Don't pay attention to the people that didn't help you." I asked him to repeat himself because I don't think my ears could believe that he was being genuine. In truth, I had never received any sage advice from the angry Italian guy ever. His words always came from a place of great hostility and rage.

After hanging up the phone on the head of the family, I called up a friend of mine, whom I like to call Big Tuna. He recently had hip surgery, and he was in Parkwood Prison but on a different floor. Big Tuna and I met during our hospital imprisonment. The Tuna is 72 years old, and he always called me up for encouragement because he was scared half to death of surgery. Via phone calls and text messages, I encouraged him to go through with both hip surgeries. He did, but he wanted to know just how come I remained very calm given I have had 15 surgeries myself. "I don't know how you do it, man," is his one-liner. He always exclaimed how extraordinary he thought I was given my scar stories.

I kindly told the Tuna, buddy, I am young, but I have so much to accomplish and I "am not even started yet. "Physically, I'm like a horse behind the racer's gate." My friend the Tuna said you should come to the third-floor complex care, the rehab is slower here, and it seems like the care team does go out of their way to provide the best possible care. I thought that if I could make that a reality, it would solve everything. If accepted on the third floor for rehab, I would have doctor malice out of my hair, and I could pay attention to rehab and get well like I'm supposed to. Now, to convince Doctor Ortho of my plans. I don't think it would be too hard to convince him that perhaps getting moved to the third floor instead of the fifth is a decision I have considered wisely.

With that in mind, I stood my ground and proclaimed to Parkwood that if they wanted me back for rehab after hip replacement surgery, then I was more than willing to participate in rehab on the third floor, and I would not compromise because I have goals, I wanted to achieve that I didn't think could have been achieved on the fifth floor because of the history and not to mention harassment.

I knew from past experiences that anytime anybody enters the hospital due to a current and or long-standing health issue; there are specific goals each patient must achieve to return safely to their home once again. So for the past few months, I refused to take NO for an answer when it came to getting what I wanted from the surgery. (Thanks, Jericho, for reminding me I still had gas left in the tank. I surveyed my plans like I was writing the table of contents for War and Peace. I was methodical, direct and very determined.

As I sat down looking to see how I could limber up like a '90's Green Power Ranger Tommy Oliver, I watched interviews via YouTube of para-sports athletes and their injuries and what made them lose their limbs. I then began to research professional wrestling injuries. Most of the injuries I researched happened to their shoulders, hips and back or biceps. I quickly realized that myself and the kids at the cool table shared scar stories. Some of their stories were very sad; others were a success. For the ones with great results, their message was the same. "DDP Yoga gave me a new lease on my career. "After several weeks of being a skeptic and just flat out procrastinating, I decided to go for it; I was 100% All in. Nothing else mattered at this point. I knew that I had a monkey on my back in the form of my cerebral palsy, and I wanted to get rid of it as best as I could. Cue the reason I titled this chapter Clark Kent's Swan Song. I suffer from Superman Syndrome. What is Superman Syndrome, you ask? It is having to always be brave in any situation. It is also an overwhelming sense to show great courage when the odds are not always in your favour. That is why I can relate to many celebrities, as funny as they may seem. Like celebrities seek tranquil moments of peace and downtime with their families when the studio lights are not bright and the cameras are not rolling. Whether your name is Denzel Washington, Adam Sandler, Mark Wallberg or even Dwayne the Rock Johnson himself, from time to time, the public must know that at the end of the day, I and the list of Hollywood stars I just named want to be normal. I have been chasing that dream for over 30 years. I am also not ashamed to admit that I will openly advocate for my health so that I can utilize resources that allow me to make progress to get back on my feet and make it the highest of priorities in my life, even if it means having to go through a 12-step labour program like Hercules. I am willing to train like a pro wrestler, meaning (no off-season), just so I can once again compete in sledge hockey and swimming and who knows, I might even try my hand at para-cycling. I would not decide to do these things for sports acclaim or medals. However, I would do it to show my nieces, Angelina, Nora, and Sianna, that you can achieve remarkable success in life no matter the obstacles or the shape or direction of your funny feet.

Acknowledgments

Sometimes when you write a book, this page is often the toughest to write because you don't want to leave anybody out who may have inspired you to continue in writing your story. As for the people I want to thank, I can name hundreds of people that deserve acclaim and to be forever attached to this book. Perhaps I wrote this book to get back at my six grade teacher Mr. Watt for not liking Italians. Maybe this autobiography has a juicy tale in between it's pages about how I challenged elementary school's biggest jock to a fight after he was caught making fun of me in fourth grade. Even though I did rough the guy up a little bit, especially during French class. I shouldn't have punched Brent in the face so many times for teasing me, but you have to forgive me because I didn't have the spirit of self-control then.

That would come later on in life.

A special shout-out request to my high school science and gym teacher, Mr. Randy Johnson or R.J. Thanks for his teaching abilities in various educational disciplines. I still know that gold on the periodic table of elements is Au. Knowing that information would come in handy during my special Olympic days in the pool, inside hockey rinks, at the bowling alleys and, yes, even at the ball diamond in my pursuit to chase that colour of medal in sports.

All kidding aside, my first set of acknowledgements is, without a doubt, the most important—the ministers or, as I affectionately call them, my three pillars of faith.

I want to thank three groups of people for making this book possible. The ministers took time out of their schedules to counsel me on physical and spiritual challenges. Your teachings and council over the years has shaped me into a man that consults with the Lord before making any life-changing decisions. The three ministers at church will forever be my three pillars of faith. That is essential because it's been their counsel and Godly wisdom that allowed me to be a person who has had the opportunity to see the fourth man, Jesus in my fiery trials of life, on more than one occasion. This continues to give me the strength and courage to run the race of faith well and not be weary.

The second group of people I would like to spotlight is the medical staff that has worked with me down through the years. Whether you are an occupational therapist or a physical therapist that helped create a rigorous exercise program for me to make a living with cerebral palsy, not only attainable but very possible.

I want to thank my surgeons, who have left scars on my hips, hamstrings, ankles, pelvis and stomach. I thank you for your tireless effort to help the sick and afflicted. As a patient of various surgeons, I had always wanted to give 120 percent when bouncing back on the road to recovery.

To the writers and editors I have been inspired by and worked with, like my journalism professor Larry Cornies, Thank you for teaching me the knowledge to make a book like this. To Chris Jericho and Mick Foley.

Your books A Lions Tale, Around the World in Spandex and Hardcore Diaries got me thinking. "Maybe, one day, before I am old and grey, I could write a book about my hardships, but before I let that idea take root in my soul, I would have to experience life firsthand and, most importantly, pray about it."

Although I have to admit that even though I have read a lot of sports biographies before Christ, not one of them came with a manual on how to write a book. Shame on you, Chris and Mr. Mick. I say that because, secretly, I have been writing this book for the past seven years, but I never felt that it was ever complete. That was until now, looking back on the writing process, I can see that as humans, we have our time and God has his. I realize that the book never felt complete until recently because I would have to go through various hardships and experiences that would allow me to build my character as a man. It is either that or God has a sense of humour. In short, God had to work the kinks out to see how much glory he could receive and the impact it could have on you, the reader.

It pays to wait on the Lord folks. It truly does.

Lastly, I would like to say a big thank you to Ardith Publishing group for believing in the concept and idea for this book. Writing and publishing a book is not easy, and the task is even more challenging during a global crisis. However, persistence and being surrounded by the right people make all the difference.

Thank you to my photographer Heather for making me photogenic. You gave the book identity, and I am truly grateful for that.

Lightning Source UK Ltd.
Milton Keynes UK
UKHW022332170223
417179UK00009B/892